Pretuel rem...

Pg 3?

D 1/2 quarts of water

THE PROTOCOL FOR HEALTH
Seven Unexpected Solutions

For Pain, Disease, Inflammation, Digestion,
Hormones, Arthritis, Fatigue, Immunity,
Autoimmunity, Weight Loss, Migraines,
Lyme Disease, and More

Written and published by
Matt Archer, D.C.

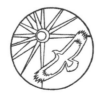

DISCLAIMER: This book is for educational purposes only. It should not be used to diagnose or treat any medical condition. For diagnosis or treatment of a medical problem, consult your physician. Before starting any diet, exercise, or health protocol consult your doctor to determine if it is appropriate for you and your circumstances. The author and publisher claim no responsibility for any adverse effects resulting from the use of information contained in this book.

Designations used by companies to distinguish their products are often claimed as trademarks. All brand names and product names used in this book and on its cover are trade names, service marks, trademarks, and registered trademarks of their respective owners. None of the companies referenced within the book have endorsed the book or the discussion of the products mentioned within.

Muscle diagrams used with permission granted by ©ICAK-U.S.A.

The Protocol for Health: Seven Unexpected Solutions
Published by Matt Archer in Nevada City, California, United States of America
contact@theprotocolforhealth.com

All rights reserved.
Copyright © 2020 by Matt Archer
Cover design and copyright © 2020 by Matt Archer
Interior book design by Stefano Landini - www.stefanolandini.com
Graphic design by Juniper Lindquist - www.juniperlindquist.com

Library of Congress Control Number: 2020922348
ISBN 978-0-578-77011-6

Printed in the United States of America

10 9 8 7 6 5 4 3 2 1
First Edition

No part of this publication may be reproduced, stored in a retrieval system, or transmitted in any form or by any means electronic, mechanical, photocopying, recording, or otherwise, without the written permission of the author/publisher.

Dedicated to life worth living for all.

Contents

- Foreword 1
- Chapter 1
  Introduction and Summary 5
  The Seven Causes of Disease 12
  The Solutions 14
- Chapter 2
  The Origin of the Seven Solutions 21
- Chapter 3
  Why Write This Book? 35

**Chapters 4 through 10
Solutions to the Seven Underlying Causes of Disease**

- Chapter 4
  Pervasive Chronic Intestinal Infection 43
  Zinc Deficiency—Intestinal Infection Flowchart 44
- Chapter 5
  Food Reactions: Allergies and Sensitivities 65
  Simple Foods Diet 77
  Cow's Milk Dairy Products 81
  Gluten 86
  Soy 90
  Corn 93
  Personal Care and Household Products 99
  Tree Nut Sensitivity 102
- Chapter 6
  Adrenal Fatigue, Blood Sugar Instability,
  and Elevated Cortisol 103
  Blood Sugar Stability - Adrenal Support Guidelines 106
  Appetite, Eating, and Absorption 112
  Intermittent Fasting? There is a Better Solution 114
- Chapter 7
  Deficiencies of Basic Vitamins and Minerals 119
  Calcium 128

Magnesium 131
B12 / B Complex / Iron 132
Major and Trace Minerals 134
Concentrated Raw Sesame Oil 135
Food-Source Vitamin A and D 136
Biost and/or Rare Red Meat 137
Zinc and Betaine Hydrochloride 138
Emerging Awareness of the Gut-Lung Axis 145

■ CHAPTER 8
Overconsumption of Carbohydrates 149
   Avoiding Illness: Colds, Influenza, Viruses, Bacteria, Etcetera 156

■ CHAPTER 9
Lack of Mild Sustained Aerobic Exercise 159
   Exercise Guidelines 164

■ CHAPTER 10
Unresolved Muscle Injuries or One-Sided Pain 169
   Neck and Upper Back Pain 170
   Shoulder Joint/Rotator Cuff Issues 172
   Low Back and Hip Pain 173
   Headaches, Migraines, and Jaw, Upper Neck, and Facial Pain 176

■ CHAPTER 11
Clearing Interference Simplifies Care 179

■ CHAPTER 12
Glands and Hormones 183
   Thyroid 185
   Adrenals 186
   Pituitary 188
   Pancreas 189
   Reproductive System/Sexual Function 191
   Female Hormone Issues and Dysmenorrhea 191
   Male Hormone Issues 195
   Problems with Blood Tests 196

- CHAPTER 13
  Solving Difficult Issues 201
  Weight Loss 201
  Inability to Gain Weight 203
  Blood Pressure 203
  Autoimmunity 204
  Rheumatoid Arthritis 204
  Multiple Sclerosis 205
  Fibromyalgia and Chronic Fatigue 205
  Carpal Tunnel and Repetitive Stress Injury 205
  Lyme Disease 206
  Migraines 206
  Narcolepsy 207
  Insomnia 207
  Addiction and Depression 209
  Anxiety, Panic, and Heartbeat Irregularities 210

- CHAPTER 14
  Solving Kids' Issues
  (Eczema, Poor Appetite, Nightmares, Frequent Illness, Etcetera) 213

- CHAPTER 15
  Athletic Performance 217

- CHAPTER 16
  Obstacles: It's Hard to Be Human 221

- ACKNOWLEDGMENTS 229

- APPENDIX A
  A Study of Cow Dairy and Low Back Pain 233

- APPENDIX B
  Resources 247

- INDEX 263

- ABOUT THE AUTHOR 279

Foreword

The challenge for me is to help you understand how, working together with my patients, we consistently resolve or reduce symptoms, pain, and disease with a protocol comprised of surprisingly simple interconnected components. While some of these solutions may be familiar, they're mostly novel in form but sensible in design. The components relating to the gut and lung microbiome offer lasting solutions to some of the most confounding and causative health issues of our time. The Protocol for Health is a whole system requiring effort and understanding. It's not a miracle supplement, juice, diet, or other one-piece cure. It's a comprehensive solution that addresses underlying causes of physical stress and creates conditions for healing and strengthening the body.

Lifelong pain is occasionally cured by a kick from a horse. There are plenty of testimonials for horse-kicking and slipping on ice, as well as supplements, juice, diets, and procedures. While testimonials can be compelling, everything has the potential to create a miracle now and then. But will a therapy work for us, and how consistently effective is it? For those answers, ideally, we look to large, expensive studies, but until those are available, we have testimonials, compelling accounts, or we try it for ourselves.

In at least the last six years since the Protocol for Health became defined, all of my adherent patients have resolved or significantly improved their conditions. But I wouldn't have believed that statement several years earlier. Consistent success with the full spectrum of health conditions seemed impossible to my skeptical self. Perhaps this book will serve as a compelling account. Ideally, you're reading now because of the success of someone you trust.

Our success comes from a breakthrough technique that reveals clear information through the body and nervous system of any patient. With this approach, patterns of muscle weakness associated with internal health issues become obvious. These issues define *seven common underlying causes of pain and disease not previously identified and addressed together.* The Protocol for Health addresses all seven causes of disease and provides solutions that have proven to be effective in practice over many years. By applying the solutions to these seven issues, people heal.

Chapter 1

Introduction and Summary

The Protocol for Health wasn't born from a theory based on secondhand ideas or learned from other sources. The Protocol revealed itself through almost twenty years of serving my patients and seeing clear patterns of muscle weakness associated with internal issues that resolve when seven causes of disease are addressed. These observations are possible because of a breakthrough in manual muscle testing that reveals these weaknesses in an obvious manner.

With this technique it is possible to identify underlying causative issues specific to a patient. While many individual pieces can be identified, the issues fall into seven *nearly universal* categories. When seven solutions are applied concurrently, people heal and become healthier and stronger. The Protocol for Health is effective throughout the healthcare spectrum at achieving more sustainable health for everyone.

The health outcomes of both mainstream and alternative healthcare are inconsistent and often inadequate, and scientific study has not managed to identify and guide the treatment of the underlying causes of most modern health issues. What is the percentage of chronic illnesses and general health issues for which modern medicine has determined the causes and solutions? I don't know, but with a little research, it's revealed that the underlying causes of most health conditions are "poorly understood" and "further research is (always) required." Heart disease is the number one killer in the U.S., which is mostly caused by arterial plaque, but what causes plaque to build up? Inflammation, maybe? We don't know. Cancer is number two and is caused by unregulated cell growth. Many contributing factors have been identified, but the cause remains uncertain. Accidents (unintentional injuries) are number three on the list, according to the Center for Disease Control. Number four is chronic lower respiratory disease. It wasn't easy to convince everyone, or to beat back the tobacco industry, but it is now established that smoking dramatically increases the risk and that breathing irritants at work is also involved. However, many people die of this condition who don't fit those categories. Number five is stroke, for which we can't identify and treat the underlying causes. Looking at the top causes of disability, there is some overlap with the above conditions, but adding arthritis, back pain, and other musculoskeletal issues, mental illness, diabetes, and nervous system disorders doesn't make us look any smarter. We don't know what causes these issues.

As for the solutions, or how to prevent these conditions from developing, we're told to eat a healthy diet, exercise, reduce stress, worry about our genes, and see our medical doctors for drugs and surgeries. Diet, exercise, and stress management are sensible routes for creating health, but the current mainstream guidelines have major blind spots and often yield poor outcomes.

What is a healthy diet? There is little agreement. We don't even have accurate laboratory testing for food allergies or sensitivities, and we certainly can't come to a consensus about ideal ratios of proteins, fats, and carbohydrates.

What is healthy exercise? There is a bit more agreement but plenty of uncertainty.

Reducing stress is nice, but it's often nearly impossible. And is emotional stress truly a primary cause of disease or could there be forms of *physical* stress that are far more important and addressable?

Advances in the field of genetics lead to announcements about the identification of disease-causing genes, but then a few years later, they walk it back and say there are important, undetermined environmental factors.

Drugs and surgeries are available as last resorts, but they don't treat causes. While it's difficult to get solid numbers, a study by Johns Hopkins Medicine found more than 250,000 people in the U.S. die *every year* from medical errors, and they have petitioned the CDC to list this as the third leading cause of death.

With accurate instant feedback from the body, it becomes clear that most people have seven foundational health issues, some of which are rarely identified and the others, rarely addressed. The solutions to these seven health issues are surprisingly simple and sensible, yet collectively, they are challenging to implement, complicated in their interconnectedness, and remarkably powerful. When these issues are addressed, dramatic improvements in the absorption of nutrients, reduction of inflammation, and elimination of chemicals and waste products from the body are achieved to a degree that I find is unprecedented in our modern environment. This heals long-term issues and improves almost every condition or pain. When these seven causative issues are treated, the full spectrum of health issues improve or resolve.

For my personal process in this, rewind twenty years to my late twenties, when my health was compromised with frequent illness, digestive problems, old injuries that wouldn't heal, and arthritis in my hands and spine. Over the years, I developed my technique and protocol piece by piece. Now, at fifty, I don't suffer from the health issues of my past, and my strength and endurance are excellent, as long as I follow the Protocol for Health. Some people don't start to lose their health until later in life, and some are born with poor health. Some seem fine until they have a heart attack. My health issues pushed me to search for solutions, and I needed a push. My search helped me realize simple solutions to restore health and how unusual it is to find those solutions and effective healthcare.

I'm not saying that I have all the answers or that we should abandon science and modern healthcare, but people often fail to recognize that science and healthcare in general are limited at creating and/or restoring health. If there is an alternative that is safe, sensible, and effective, isn't it worth a try?

Your willingness to try, and to achieve the possibility of health, is what matters. Without health, nothing works. If you can prove to yourself that the Protocol for Health is effective, you can maintain a better quality of life, the ability to do what you love, and the ability to care for those whom you love for longer. Once you know it works, then you know there is a route forward and a solution for the health issues of your loved ones. Some will need to wait for science to support my claims with large studies, but if people lead the way by consistently resolving their symptoms and health issues, science and medicine will follow.

People who practice the Protocol consistently achieve excellent results with inflammation, chronic pain, old injuries, chronic illness, digestive issues, hormone imbalance, autoimmune conditions, migraines, allergies, headaches, hypersensitivity, skin conditions, chronic fatigue, fibromyalgia, endocrine issues, etcetera. These claims sound far-fetched, but with honesty and confidence, this is what I tell my new patients because if they follow the Protocol, within two months of starting care, they see that it works. After another four or five months, their health issues are usually resolved.

Understand this is not a protocol that has been scientifically established beyond my practice for treating any disease or the long list of conditions above. This is a protocol for health. *It's about removing obstacles so the body can heal itself.* People should see medical doctors to rule out diseases or conditions that could be immediately life-threatening. Even when symptoms disappear, they should work with medical doctors to determine whether or not one has a disease to treat. While the recovery of health that we see with this protocol is remarkable, of course there are limitations. Some tissues can heal, and some can't. Structural changes or deformities can be obstacles to full resolution of pain. There can also be a point at which people can be too sick, tired, old, or confused to manage this regimen; otherwise, it's inspiring to see what people can heal and how many issues can be resolved.

Within at least the last six years of practice, I can say with confidence that every patient who has followed the Protocol has seen significant improvement or resolution of symptoms. While there are many conditions I don't claim to treat, I guide patients in a system that enables them to become stronger and healthier and attain better nutrient absorption, waste product elimination, and less inflammation.

Is there any condition that wouldn't benefit from these components? While almost all health issues improve with these pieces, established cancer may or may not fit in that category. I don't know how to treat cancer. The key is not to get it in the first place. Cancer involves unregulated cell growth the body cannot identify as a problem. If we help a body to be stronger and absorb better, does it enable the immune system to step up and fight off cancer? We can't know the answer, but it must depend on the type of cancer, how far it's progressed, and many other factors.

What I do know is how to help people become stronger, how to restore a healthy appetite, strengthen the immune system, improve energy, sleep better, eliminate toxins, clear muscle weakness, and reduce inflammation and pain. All of these pieces are factors in the prevention of cancer and may be tremendously valuable to someone going through cancer treatments and dealing with the associated side effects.

The overall results achieved by mainstream and alternative medicine with most pain, disease, and other complaints are highly inconsistent. Patients are often disappointed with the outcome of care and aren't given a sensible route forward to a long-term solution. If a technique, supplement, or drug can be proven to be just slightly more effective than a placebo, then medical doctors, influencers, vendors, and the public are on board even though it's only slightly effective. Many drugs, supplements, and surgical procedures that are clinically proven effective are only slightly more effective than a placebo. In a field where causes and real solutions are rarely determined, something proven to be slightly effective looks pretty good in comparison.

Unfortunately, studies on chiropractic and acupuncture show underwhelming results as well. That doesn't mean those approaches don't work, or that people don't receive great benefit from these modalities. It means sometimes they work and sometimes they don't, and usually, the results fall somewhere in between. If you received a miracle solution from the right chiropractic adjustment or the right acupuncture treatment, then it may come as a surprise that on average these techniques work only slightly better than a placebo. If you know you can control or eliminate your low back pain with yoga, "core-strengthening" exercises, or chiropractic adjustments you may wonder why everyone doesn't just do that. These modalities don't work for everyone. If however, you have worked with multiple practitioners and specialists without success, or been told the problem is in your head, or you are just getting old, or that you will have to keep coming back for endless new treatments, supplements, herbs, drugs, or surgeries, then you may have already discovered for yourself that established healthcare rarely treats the causes of disease.

For a healthcare regimen to work consistently it must address all of the main components of an issue at their cause. Significant chronic or recurring pain or disease is rarely caused by one simple factor. If it was, established healthcare would get better results. It may be that accurate instant feedback through the nervous system that is specific to an individual is the only way to identify and address multiple causative issues. When you achieve this kind of feedback, it becomes apparent that **most people are dealing with the same seven main factors that cumulatively cause most health issues, pain, and disease.** When these issues are simultaneously addressed, consistent, excellent results can be achieved with the full spectrum of symptoms and conditions.

I'm a second-generation chiropractor who took a skeptical approach to a popular but controversial chiropractic technique called applied kinesiology. Over the past twenty years of study and practice, I've developed a breakthrough protocol that builds on that technique and an innovative form of manual muscle testing that guides patients to effective solutions. I primarily utilize diet, exercise, lifestyle, simple supplements, and myofascial muscle work. I use traditional or modified chiropractic adjustments when indicated and only when a patient wants them for accelerated relief of symptoms. Patients don't have to be adjusted with force to achieve a solution. The Protocol for Health also incorporates aspects of functional medicine, Ayurveda, traditional Chinese medicine, cranial-sacral therapy, and other modalities. The unifying principle of my practice is simplification. Low-carb Paleo and ketogenic diets and the principles of Ancestral Health support choosing simple forms of diet, exercise, and supplements. My technique of manual muscle testing yields clear, instantaneous feedback through a patient's nervous system so that weaknesses and clear solutions, specific to the patient, are quickly determined with an exceptional level of clarity. Before developing this method and observing the results for myself, my family, friends, and patients, I never imagined there could be a health solution that works for so many conditions but consists of such basic components.

I developed this technique and protocol through academic study and clinical work that integrates and builds on the work of many innovative doctors. My perspective is informed by explorations of limits and boundaries in kinesiology, mechanics, mountain sports, machinery, yoga, meditation, and other physical and spiritual practices. Thirteen years ago, my focus shifted more to family, health, home, and livelihood with my wife and daughters, who truly have become my most essential teachers. I combine skeptic and mystic, science and spirituality. These contradictions lead me to look for strong, clear answers in a wide variety of fields. I believe my technique is teachable and reproducible but determining that will require studies and/or the experience of many more people learning, guiding, and practicing this modality. In the meantime, I offer simple solutions that are surprisingly effective.

The Protocol for Health addresses the following components. Most people have, or will have, compromised health from all of these:

THE SEVEN CAUSES OF DISEASE

1. **Chronic intestinal infection**, a pathogen established in the gut, that may or may not cause digestive symptoms and is usually allowed into the body by weak stomach acid that is caused by zinc deficiency, physical stress, and inadequate nutrition.

2. **Food reactions** (allergies and sensitivities) that go unrecognized because of continual exposure to these foods, the complication of chronic intestinal infection, and the established inability of laboratory testing to accurately determine food allergies and sensitivities.
3. **Blood sugar instability** because of excessive caffeine and/or activity on an empty stomach, weak appetite, and/or inadequate or infrequent protein consumption.
4. **Deficiencies of simple nutrients** because we don't eat what we were designed to eat, modern food is compromised, most supplements are poorly utilized, and most of us have weak stomach acid and intestinal infection that interfere with absorption.
5. **Overconsumption of carbohydrates** because of the advent of agriculture and our love of sugar—fruit, grain, legumes, potatoes, and any other form of sugar or starch.
6. **Lack of sustained mild aerobic exercise** because we drive cars, but we were designed to walk for transportation. Short trips or even repeated short trips do not adequately strengthen the heart.
7. **Unresolved muscle injuries** because weakness and deficiencies from the previous six components make us vulnerable and interfere with healing.

I find these seven components to be the primary causes of most health issues and disease.

While this book explains the process of addressing these issues, in some cases it would be dangerous to attempt to put these pieces together without the guidance and feedback of a qualified doctor or practitioner. This book can't be a complete how-to guide because some aspects of the Protocol require in-person guidance, not only for the safety of some patients, but also to identify muscle weaknesses, reflex points, reactions to foods, old muscle injuries, etcetera. However, for most people of average health, the components of the Protocol are safe and simple and have great potential.

With a few simple supplements and the guidelines herein, people have access to a powerful health solution. While the pieces are safe and simple, a doctor should be consulted before starting any new health program. People also need to pay attention to how they feel in the process. If any piece of the Protocol causes discomfort or significant issues, it should be discontinued, and professional guidance should be found. It would be ideal to work with a doctor familiar with this approach. It is likely that, before long, others will offer the Protocol for Health. This method of muscle testing may be the only system of accurate, instantaneous feedback that is specific to a patient for revealing causative health issues.

First, the short version of the solutions to each of the seven main causes. The solutions are explored in detail in Chapters 4 through 10.

THE SOLUTIONS

1. Eliminate Chronic Intestinal Infection and Address Its Cause

Chronic intestinal infection is perhaps the most common and problematic health issue affecting most people, which is almost never effectively treated and even less often with lasting results. Resolving intestinal infection is much easier than people realize, and it allows the other six factors to yield full benefits. It is an effective alternative to the usual attempts to support, rebalance, or build up beneficial gut flora or the microbiota. Chronic intestinal infection can be cleared in twenty days with specific digestive enzymes taken three times per day and away from food. Most digestive enzyme supplements are used to compensate for weak digestion, but this part of the Protocol is about breaking down and digesting the defensive structures of the intestinal infection. This is usually a comfortable process if combined with a good, simple diet and sometimes with additional supplements or support for the liver and gallbladder.

Once intestinal infection is cleared, its recurrence can usually be prevented by taking an *absorbable* zinc supplement that can be *more fully utilized*. This involves also supplementing with betaine hydrochloride, or stomach acid in a pill, because zinc is difficult or impossible to fully absorb without strong stomach acid, and it is essential for making stomach acid. This combination of digesting away intestinal infection and preventing its recurrence by strengthening stomach acid is the revolutionary foundation of this protocol, and these pieces affect all health conditions.

Zinc absorption, stomach acid production, and digestion in general are compromised by stress and stress-related hormones. However, *physical stress* more than emotional stress is the main driver of these hormones. The primary physical stresses to compromise digestion are the seven causes of disease. While emotional stress clearly makes underlying issues worse and contributes to weak stomach acid, it's not the primary driver of physical symptoms, which becomes apparent when physical stresses are resolved.

Absorbing zinc in a usable form is more difficult than people realize, and zinc is needed for stomach acid production. This is the essential foundation for preventing the recurrence of intestinal infection and food poisoning. Strong stomach acid kills pathogens before they can reach the intestines and is necessary for absorbing nutrients effectively.

2. Avoid Common Food Irritants

Most people with negative physical symptoms don't realize they are constantly reacting to some, or all, of the common subsidized foods in the U.S.: corn, cow's milk dairy products, soy, and wheat or gluten in general. I usually recommend patients eliminate these foods for at least two months while the other pieces of the Protocol are put into place. If intestinal infection isn't cleared at the same time, many will fail to benefit from removing these foods from the diet. For example, if a patient has previously tried a gluten-free or dairy-free diet but saw no benefit, I recommend they try it again during and after the process of clearing intestinal infection. Eliminating dairy and gluten from the diet is much easier than eliminating corn and soy because corn and soy are used to make most additives, synthetic vitamins, and preservatives, and they are in most prepared foods, supplements, and personal care products.

My patients who follow the Protocol find that by two months into the process, or earlier, their physical symptoms are diminished or eliminated, but they see their symptoms return from eating the common food irritants. In this way, patients discover they've been reacting to these foods constantly but were unaware. After about six months of following the Protocol, reactions to these foods decrease, and it is possible that they can be consumed occasionally without recreating symptoms.

3. Stabilize Blood Sugar

Blood sugar instability is the primary cause of adrenal fatigue, elevated cortisol, ligament laxity, inability to sleep for eight hours, and most knee pain. These issues usually resolve when people consistently eat protein at breakfast and don't go more than three hours without protein in the busy part of their day. Caffeine, sugar, and alcohol are best consumed in moderation, only right after protein, and never on an empty stomach. Despite the many long, complicated, or impossible regimens said to heal the adrenals, it really is this simple. Alas, coffee alone doesn't count as breakfast.

4. Eat and Absorb Simple Nutrients
Deficiencies of basic vitamins and minerals is a universal issue. Zinc is the most important deficiency because it's essential for stomach acid production. Weak stomach acid decreases the absorption of all vitamins and minerals, including zinc, and it allows pathogens, such as yeast, bacteria, protozoa, parasites, and viruses to survive the stomach acid and make their home in the intestines, creating chronic intestinal infection. Intestinal infection can severely impact the absorption of vitamins, minerals, and other nutrients and leads to an enormous variety of conditions including liver and gallbladder issues, poor hormone regulation, osteoporosis, anemia, heartbeat irregularities, panic attacks, and back pain, to name a few.

A study in *The Lancet* medical journal shows that increased atmospheric carbon dioxide (CO_2) decreases the ability of plants to uptake zinc and a few other minerals. This means all of us, including people living in the middle of the Amazon and the deer in our backyard, don't get as much zinc from our diets as we did before industrialization.

Almost twenty years of research and development of my protocol and system of muscle testing reveals that nearly everyone is zinc deficient and therefore has weak stomach acid, which results in intestinal infection and the associated issues. I believe the main drivers of this deficiency are atmospheric changes, compromised diet, and elevated cortisol, which suppress digestion and the ability to make effective stomach acid.

So far, modern medicine has failed to enable effective absorption of calcium supplements, but I find zinc is more difficult to absorb in a form we can fully utilize. Without fully absorbing zinc, stomach acid production is compromised as is our ability to absorb *zinc,* calcium, B12, and the other essential vitamins and minerals. Just because laboratory work shows the presence of a particular nutrient in our blood doesn't mean it can be utilized in the tissues where it is needed. When people more fully absorb nutrients in usable forms, the results are obvious in terms of resolution of symptoms, increases in strength, and improvements in certain blood tests. My patients consistently confirm they feel noticeably better when absorption is addressed and they take carefully chosen, mostly food-based supplements. Healthcare in general remains unaware of how powerful simple food-based supplements can be because supplements are almost never adequately absorbed and utilized.

Most vitamin and mineral supplements are made from rocks, food irritants, and chemicals and have little to no value. Even high-end multivitamins contain corn and soy and synthetic pseudo-vitamins. Supplements are part of the cause of negative symptoms for most people who take them, and even the best quality supplements are *minimally absorbed* because of the underlying conditions of weak stomach acid and chronic intestinal infection. It's difficult to find supplements that achieve great results. With instant accurate feedback through a patient's nervous system, carefully selected, mostly food-sourced supplements, and a good simple diet, health issues can be treated at their cause.

The chain of events that leads from zinc deficiency to chronic intestinal infection, and the associated symptoms, are summarized in a flow chart on page 44. This chart outlines what I see as the cause and solution of the most universal and unrecognized underlying health issue of our time.

5. Avoid Excess Carbohydrates

When weak stomach acid and intestinal infection are addressed, low-carb Paleo and ketogenic diets consistently work very well for those who are willing to reduce carbohydrate consumption. The Paleo diet is an attempt to approximate what our ancestors ate before the advent of agriculture. Mostly it entails limiting the intake of carbohydrates, sugar, and starch, such as grains, legumes, potatoes, fruit, and any form of sugar from honey to corn syrup. It's also about carefully avoiding many food additives that are in most prepared foods. The diet consists mainly of meat, eggs, vegetables, and possibly moderate quantities of nuts and fruit. I find that goat dairy products may be included by most people, but the large proteins in cow dairy products, or alpha S1 casein, can be demonstrated to cause weakness and inflammation for most people.

6. Walking or Sustained Mild Aerobic Exercise
Humans started walking less when we invented agriculture, and much less with the invention of automobiles, and now most of us in the U.S. don't walk except for short trips. Mild sustained exercise such as walking strengthens the heart without stressing it. Many people think walking at work, or repeated short trips, or taking lots of steps throughout the day has the same benefits as continuous walking, but it doesn't. Walking continuously for at least thirty to forty minutes, four to six times per week, or doing some form of repetitive exercise that approximates this type of activity, is essential to health. The key is to mildly elevate the heart rate with sustained movement. Most people either don't exercise, exercise too hard, or work primarily on their skeletal muscles and not on the heart and lungs. Considering heart disease is the number one killer in the U.S., it makes sense to focus on the heart and lungs first and then work on skeletal muscle after an aerobic foundation has been established. This isn't only a route to health, longevity, and less pain but also how some of the top modern athletes rose to success.

7. Resolve Residual Muscle Injuries

With the previous six factors in place, most old injuries heal spontaneously, but sometimes extra attention is needed, or an accelerated resolution of pain may be reason to initiate this process earlier in care. It's possible to identify residual muscle injuries by manually testing all of the main muscles that cross an area of pain or discomfort to identify any remaining muscle weaknesses. Muscle injuries usually present with pain on one side of the body, and the pain is usually opposite the weak muscle that was initially injured. My technique can be used to clear the injury by determining whether the solution is myofascial muscle work, a nutritional factor, or an energetic component. Most residual muscle injuries involve one or more of these three components and can be cleared quickly. In this manner, old patterns of pain, weakness, and imbalance can be addressed efficiently and with lasting results.

★★★

The first three chapters of this book discuss the background for the development of the Protocol for Health. Chapters 4 through 10 explore the seven main causes of disease and their solutions. Chapters 11 through 15 discuss specific conditions, their solutions, and athletic performance. Chapter 16 considers the obstacles to the Protocol for Health.

Chapter 2
Origin of the Seven Solutions

By taking a different approach to the manual muscle testing system of applied kinesiology and developing a breakthrough that builds on that method, I have created an extraordinarily effective healthcare protocol. In the process, the field of muscle testing has gone from subtle or confusing to clear and reproducible. It's possible to see obvious and instantaneous changes in muscle strength when patients taste foods or supplements or touch reflex points on the body that cause positive or negative reactions. This modality uses a person's nervous system to get accurate, instantaneous feedback about weaknesses and their potential solutions. Because muscle testing of this type has not been established as a medically objective tool, I don't call any of these pieces a diagnosis. However, the consistent results we achieve, combined with the fact that my adherent patients always confirm the accuracy of the muscle testing for themselves, leaves us with no doubt about the legitimacy of this system. The Protocol makes it possible to consistently achieve results beyond anything I or my patients have previously experienced.

Here, I describe how I developed the Protocol so that you have some understanding of how I work with my patients and how I came to these solutions. To follow the Protocol, one doesn't need to experience or understand muscle testing. But gaining some insight into the *interface of muscle weakness associated with certain organ or glandular issues* is helpful for considering how a different form of healthcare is possible. If you recognize the limitations of laboratory testing, massive studies, and mainstream and alternative medicine to create positive health outcomes, then you may be open to a form of healthcare that obtains clear information through a person's nervous system.

When I first studied applied kinesiology in a one hundred-hour course, I found it to be remarkable but also confusing and subtle. While there are applied kinesiology practitioners known to achieve excellent results with patients, the system has not been proven to be accurate or reproducible. It seemed to me, it would be helpful to first establish a clear baseline for testing and to establish the difference between weak and strong with any muscle before trying to use the testing to identify more complicated weakness, injury, sensitivity, or deficiency. It took several years to determine how to consistently, temporarily weaken a previously strong muscle for the purpose of comparison. Achieving this predictable weakening not only reveals a clear baseline, but it also removes uncertainty from testing and helps to reveal foundational health issues and their solutions.

With my system of testing, it becomes apparent that everyone weakens while they touch and hold a reflex point between the eyebrows when certain interfering factors have been resolved. There are eight possible interfering factors, which I won't describe here, but when these are addressed, any semi-isolated muscle that previously tested strong, will weaken while a person keeps a finger on this reflex point. It's unknown why people weaken to this point, but it's obvious and predictable under these conditions. At an initial visit with a patient, it takes a couple minutes to temporarily clear the factors that interfere with this reflex. After one or two follow-up appointments, most patients who continue to follow the Protocol will always test weak when they hold this point, indicating that the interfering factors have been resolved.

Once patients weaken to this reflex point, it is easy to feel the difference in strength between a muscle that is strong or weak (neurologically facilitated or inhibited). While this comparison is obvious in big, strong patients, it can be somewhat subtle with smaller patients. Having this reflex available, allows us to recheck and compare strong versus weak at any time during a visit so that uncertainty can be resolved. Seeing this clear change in strength also confirms that we are obtaining clear testing through a patient's nervous system, and it can be helpful for patients to observe instant, obvious, and predictable changes in strength in a variety of muscles throughout the body.

My technique doesn't rely on subtle changes in timing, which is the key to applied kinesiology (AK) and other systems of manual muscle testing. I'm testing for obvious changes in the simple physical strength of semi-isolated muscles of the patient. While testing, I wait to feel that a patient is pushing firmly before I increase pressure to test their strength. While it looks essentially the same as conventional AK muscle testing, it is quite different. My testing is slightly slower and reduces the possibility of jumping the gun or testing a patient's strength before they are ready and able to apply full force. While the subtle changes in timing that AK and most systems of manual muscle testing rely upon may detect certain changes in the nervous system and may yield useful therapies, I find that clearer answers lead to bigger, simpler solutions that address causative issues and consistently resolve almost all health issues.

The change in strength of a patient's semi-isolated muscle with my system of testing is often the difference of less than a pound of pressure demonstrating weakness to muscles that can't be overpowered with forty to eighty pounds of pressure. When muscle testing is this clear, false answers are mostly eliminated, and there is always a means to double-check the sensitivity of testing.

Here and on the cover, I've included a link to a video demonstration of this testing.

www.theprotocolforhealth.com/video
or

In the video, I demonstrate clear changes in muscle strength with a big, strong person on the table. The testing is also clear, although less so for an outside observer, when testing smaller people.

Each of the solutions of the Protocol relates to a specific muscle weakness, which is part of how I originally identified their significance. By referring to the works of the founders of applied kinesiology and looking to simple, sensible solutions, I've identified components that help patients resolve all of the normal weaknesses we come across. Most of the diagrams I've included are the muscles I find weak in most patients. A few diagrams are included to illustrate muscles that are often tight or painful when compensating for common weaknesses. In general, not all of the weaknesses are apparent at the same time or at the beginning of care, but over the course of a few weeks or a few office visits, these weaknesses can be identified and resolved.

During a typical office visit, we test a couple dozen components relating to a patient's health. The answers are specific to the patient and come through their nervous system. When the indicated therapy is applied, clear results are achieved such that a patient can challenge them on their own, or with medical supervision if necessary, and confirm the relevance to their symptoms. People see the results with reduced symptoms and improved health, quality of life, and objective findings: blood count, vitamin and mineral blood levels, inflammatory markers, blood pressure, cholesterol levels, bone density, lung capacity, grip strength, pH of saliva and urine, range of motion, gained muscle mass, body fat reduction, etcetera.

At follow-up visits, mostly with muscle testing, we check many components: zinc absorption and stomach acid production, other vitamin or mineral deficiencies, presence or absence of intestinal infection, blood sugar stability or adrenal fatigue, excess carbohydrate consumption, food reactions, allergen exposure, appropriate exercise level, acute viral or bacterial infections, the need for myofascial muscle work to clear unresolved injuries, and other factors.

This system of testing is sensitive and accurate enough to demonstrate that, for people with the particular food sensitivity, ingesting cow's milk proteins weakens muscles of core strength and contributes to low back pain; corn weakens a muscle in the rotator cuff of the shoulder and may also cause tennis elbow; repeatedly drinking coffee on an empty stomach stresses the adrenal glands, which weakens three associated muscles that cross the knee and often leads to pain and instability, and a variety of other clear connections that could be proven with clinical studies.

By following up with people in the office we get to see the effective application of, or lack of compliance with, the above pieces of this protocol.

With this clarity added to the technique of applied kinesiology, it becomes obvious that the foundation of that system can give remarkable insight into patterns of muscle weakness associated with pain and disease. The muscle-organ/gland association which the founder of applied kinesiology, Dr. George Goodheart, discovered in the 1960s, and which is taught by the International College of Applied Kinesiology (ICAK), can give tremendous insight when used in a clear manner. By first establishing a baseline for muscle testing—the essential foundation of my technique—a clear correlation between the strength of a muscle and the state of health of its associated organ or gland can be observed.

Some examples of the muscle-organ/gland association are the relationships of the psoas major muscles to the kidneys, a portion of the pectoralis muscles with the liver, and the teres minor muscles with the thyroid. These correlations relate to the meridian system used in traditional Chinese medicine and Ayurveda. When testing is clear, it's easy to demonstrate that weakness of the same muscle

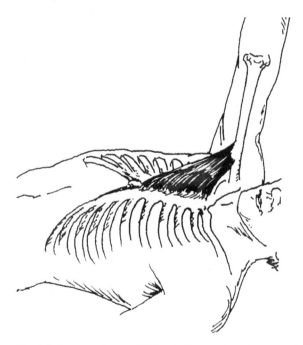

1. Pectoralis Major — Sternal Head. From the chest to the upper arm.

on both sides of the body (bilateral muscle weakness), is usually caused by stress or weakness of the associated organ or gland.

For example, there's a link between stress to the liver and pain in the upper back, shoulder, neck, and/or tension headaches. When the liver is stressed, the sternal head of the pectoralis major muscle will be weak (Figure 1 previous page), which causes tension in the opposing upper trapezii muscles (Figure 2 below) of the upper back, neck, and base of the skull. This tension is an automatic compensation to partially balance or stabilize a compromised joint. The compensation often causes muscle spasms and pain. Rubbing the tight upper trapezii only offers temporary relief. When liver stress is resolved, full strength returns to the chest, and pain and tension in the upper trapezii decrease. This outcome is predictable, even with patients who've had upper back pain for fifty years and were certain it was caused by stress,

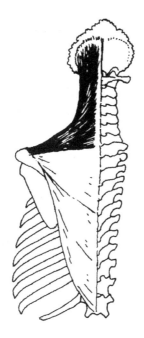

2. Trapezius — Upper Division. From the skull and neck to the shoulder.

employment, hormones, or an old injury. The solution is not just another temporary liver cleanse but clearing the cause of liver congestion by eliminating chronic intestinal infection. There are many such examples of opposing tension causing pain because of muscle weakness associated with stressed organs or glands, some of which are described later. Again, these associations were identified by the founders of applied kinesiology, but without a clear baseline for testing, these associations were often quite subtle.

When I demonstrate this form of testing for teachers of the ICAK, they suggest I'm testing something different and that it could be problematic or misleading. It is different. While it took a few years to consistently, temporarily weaken a strong muscle for comparison, this predictable change in strength is essential for establishing a clear baseline and observing obvious changes in muscle strength. Under these conditions, many of the known problems and overly complicated components of AK are resolved. The problems of neurologic disorganization, "switching," and muscles that don't weaken in a predictable manner, which are described in the texts of applied kinesiology, are resolved with this form of testing. With these advances, the ICAK or others could prove accuracy, reproducibility, and interexaminer reliability in manual muscle testing.

Many doctors, practitioners, and laypeople use AK and other systems of manual muscle testing in a variety of ways for answers about reactions to foods, supplements, therapies, and more esoteric questions. Sometimes these approaches yield positive outcomes for patients, but often they're ineffective or require an endless string of new supplements, therapies, and return visits. When muscle testing is made to be clearer, it becomes possible to identify causative issues rather than treating peripheral components.

Many people are familiar with systems of muscle testing that involve testing one's self or testing other people to vials of foods, supplements, irritants, or other things held in hand or placed on the body. I think those forms of testing fall into the categories of intuitive or energetic testing. By instead working with sense of taste, reflex points, and clear changes in muscle strength, it's possible to get clearer answers about causative issues that are rarely thrown off by interfering factors. Some practitioners of other systems of muscle testing describe interference in test results from components such as a change in the label adhesive used by the manufacturer of test bottles, or a phone in a pocket, competing intentions, or having a bad day. I don't find these problems. While it would be more convenient to have people hold vials rather than taste foods and supplements, holding vials of possible irritants or solutions creates no change in strength within my system of testing. While testing to items held in hand may be useful for some, it's not part of the curriculum of the ICAK, it defies explanation through known neurologic pathways, and it doesn't seem as if it could be proven to be objective. I'm not saying it can't be done, I just think this is a better and more direct method of testing.

This book describes a path for consistently addressing causes of muscle weakness, pain, and disease that continue to baffle mainstream and alternative medicine. Consider low back pain, which is suffered by more than 80 percent of adults in the U.S. at some point in their lives. Most sources don't want to talk about the fact that the cause of 85 percent of low back pain can't be determined, let alone successfully treated. No established low back pain treatments work consistently. Perhaps even more alarming is that the prevalence of chronic low back pain is rapidly increasing. A 2009 study in the Archives of Internal Medicine reported that the prevalence of chronic low back pain more than doubled during a fourteen-year study, and other sources confirm the increase in disability and the associated burden on healthcare.

All of my patients of the last several years with chronic low back pain have significantly reduced or eliminated their pain with the Protocol. While my system of testing reveals several contributing factors, low back pain is most clearly associated with chronic intestinal infection. For some time, I thought the reaction to cow's milk proteins was the biggest factor. Then I realized that chronic intestinal infection was either becoming more common or easier to identify. Intestinal infection and dairy consumption create similar patterns of muscle weakness.

While it can't be known with certainty, and diagnosis and tracking of the related issues are limited, it seems chronic intestinal infection has become significantly more common over the last thirty years. I think the increased prevalence of chronic intestinal infection is the cause of increased prevalence of low back pain, reactions to foods, digestive problems, chronic pain, autoimmunity, most issues relating to the gut and lung microbiome, and the overall decline of health in the U.S. and throughout the world. I find clearing intestinal infection to be an essential component of consistently improving or resolving the above conditions.

As for low back pain, what if the main cause is weakness of the psoas major muscles (Figure 3 next page) that causes the opposing tension and pain in the low back? The psoai are the primary muscles of core strength that attach to T12 through L5 and the intervertebral discs of the low back. What if the primary causes of this weakness are chronic intestinal infection, reaction to milk proteins, vitamin A deficiency, and dehydration? That could be proven if one knew how to consistently clear chronic intestinal infection and test people to vitamin A supplements to establish that supplements containing corn and soy should be avoided by most patients. And what if most conditions and pain had similar explanations that could be cleared with diet and mostly food-based supplements? Well, they do, and they can be, and it's easy

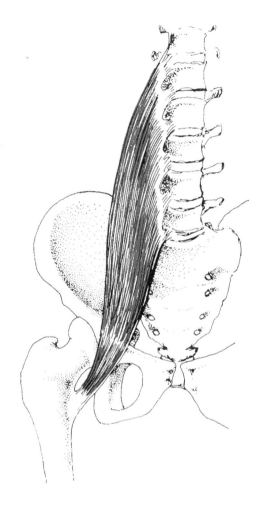

3. Psoas Major. From the spine to the femur.

to demonstrate with a system that yields accurate feedback from the body.

By establishing a clear baseline for this testing, weaknesses identified with manual muscle testing become remarkably obvious. While there may be a few different reasons for a particular muscle weakness, with this system it's relatively easy to determine the cause of the weakness and clear it. For the example of low back pain, the weak psoas muscles can be identified, and the founders of applied kinesiology established that the psoas relates to the kidneys by way of the acupuncture meridians. Any significant stress to the kidneys can cause weakness of the related psoai, which causes the opposing tension and possible pain in the low back. Dehydration, vitamin A deficiency, cow's milk proteins, and intestinal infection can all stress the kidneys. Once these factors are addressed, this technique makes it possible to identify if there is an additional cause of weakness of the psoai, such as calcium deficiency, an old muscle injury, or an issue stemming from the feet. These and other issues associated with the low back can then be resolved more easily and effectively because the issues related to the kidneys were addressed first, which cleared the bilateral weakness of the psoas.

This example above illustrates the multiple components requiring some knowledge, skill, and management to resolve, but with three to six office visits over the course of as many weeks, it's possible to address the factors related to low back pain and show a person how to keep them from returning. If we could only do that much, it would be revolutionary, but clearing these issues affects much more than just the low back. The "incidental side effects" could be clearing the cause of anemia, osteoporosis, IBS, restless leg, and terrible menstrual cycles or other seemingly unconnected symptoms that are actually closely associated.

One of the most remarkable things to demonstrate at a follow-up visit is whether a person sensitive to corn or cow's milk proteins has consumed either in the few days before an appointment. Both of these foods, and in some cases soy as well, can create a specific pattern of muscle weakness that reveals a patient's sensitivity to these foods and confirms their recent consumption of that food. It's a great opportunity in care for people to see the sensitivity and accuracy of muscle testing. The news of exposure to these foods may come as a surprise to the patient, and they may deny consuming it, but further conversation may help them realize a component they had been unaware of, such as milk chocolate containing milk proteins, or that a little parmesan cheese creates an obvious pattern of weakness, or that citric acid (usually made from corn) in their toothpaste is enough to weaken a specific shoulder muscle and cause mental fog, a rash, and/or general inflammation.

This feedback about particular reactions to foods is often helpful for motivating patients to take steps to avoid these food irritants. Removing the problematic food(s) from the diet, they see the reduction of pain and inflammation or other symptoms; but consuming the food causes symptoms to return. Constantly observing this process in practice has made it apparent to me and my patients that reactions to the four main subsidized foods create significant symptoms far more often than is realized. Most people with health issues react to some or all of these foods, and they cause surprisingly significant issues. But simply eliminating the offending foods is often not enough to see the benefits. The food reactions and the ability to reduce those reactions are usually complicated by intestinal infection, elevated cortisol, and the rest of the seven factors.

By clearing the seven main causes of disease, addressing muscle weaknesses, and making sure a patient has a handle on how to keep it that way, people heal. Frequently, they eliminate lifelong issues or significant complaints related to the full spectrum of mild to dangerous health conditions.

My hope is that this information will inspire others to try and to benefit from these solutions so people realize healthcare can be much simpler and more effective than what we thought was possible. There really are just seven main causes of disease. Yes, there will still be infectious disease and chemical exposure, but these seven solutions address a large portion of why some people pass easily through those experiences and others have severe reactions. When the seven issues are addressed, inflammation decreases, absorption of nutrients increases, elimination of chemicals and excess hormones improves, the immune system strengthens, muscle weaknesses clear, opposing tension and pain resolve, and sleep, energy, and overall health improve.

Chapter 3

Why Write This Book?

Why write this book? Because it's the right thing to do, and everyone should have access to an effective healthcare solution. I like to think that if I share my observations and discoveries, then they will spread in a good way. These solutions work too well to be kept and not shared. How sweet it would be if sharing and implementing these ideas were a watershed moment in healthcare!

I am asking people to think about health differently and to try solutions that are unexpected. Developing and communicating the Protocol has definitely had its challenges. My process of developing the Protocol started twenty years ago as I questioned my teacher of the ICAK. It wasn't until about six years ago that it was apparent that all patients who were able to completely follow the Protocol achieved excellent results. Still, not all patients are willing to follow the entire system, even though a two-month trial often leads to the transformation of an individual's health. It's certainly more than I can explain in a single office visit, and not everyone is open to trying something new. For those willing to read this book, it goes a long way in explaining how this system was developed, how to follow it, and why it works.

When a carpenter comes to me with low back pain and I suggest he eliminate cow dairy products from his diet and take digestive enzymes three times per day between meals for twenty days to clear an intestinal infection he may not realize he has, you can see the difficulty of the conversation. To make it worse, I'm a chiropractor who is supposed to deliver chiropractic adjustments. If I can't confirm the need for a traditional chiropractic adjustment, that carpenter may be disappointed by non-force adjustments while we clear the muscle weaknesses caused by internal issues that create the subluxations chiropractors adjust. He may walk out the door thinking I did nothing more than yammer on about some protocol and long-term, system-wide solution, when all he came for was an "adjustment" to his low back. If he isn't aware of other symptoms, and only has low back pain occasionally, and isn't interested in working on his overall health, this approach appears as an unnecessary, slow, expensive hassle compared to "Hey, doc, pop my back." Unfortunately, just popping his back does carry some risk, and studies suggest it only works a little better than a placebo. Of course, the right chiropractic adjustment that creates an apparent miracle and allows the patient to jump up off the table is always excellent when you get it.

The Protocol for Health is not an instant fix. Two months or less is quick when it comes to clearing a chronic issue, but for an acute episode of low back pain that usually clears in about a week, it may not be worth it. However, this approach still has a decent chance of providing instant relief, and when people want to stop having *recurring* episodes of low back pain or are ready to address a *chronic* issue, I can virtually guarantee results if they follow this process and come in for a handful of follow-up appointments.

The Protocol requires that people try something different

from what they've been doing, and different from what almost everyone is doing. Going against the tide requires self-discipline, patience, and persistence. That may be too much to ask if symptoms are mild and infrequent and if people have already determined that health is a crap-shoot, nothing really works, it's all determined by genetics and stress, they'll just have to live with it, or wait until their condition is bad enough for drugs or surgery or some miracle therapy.

But who goes to a chiropractor for bad digestive issues, hormonal complaints, skin conditions, or the myriad of other symptoms I frequently help people resolve? It's challenging to be a chiropractor who doesn't perform many traditional chiropractic adjustments and who borrows from an unproven technique called applied kinesiology that has profound components and blind spots. When people go to a chiropractor, they expect to lie back and receive a treatment, not to be told they can transform their health and their medical future, and they have to do most of the work themselves.

I was in practice over ten years before I could virtually guarantee results with the Protocol. There were several years when I helped people accurately identify food reactions, but I didn't recognize the pervasive nature of chronic intestinal infection and how it complicates those reactions. In the past, some patients achieved excellent results from eliminating certain foods from the diet and implementing the rest of this system before it was fully developed, but others, not so much. The effort and expense for some was not rewarded with success, and it was easy to feel I had failed these people. It has been a process over the years that taught me that any of the seven factors can create an obstacle to the resolution of symptoms. It also took time to understand how to differentiate between concrete physical weaknesses, relevant reflex points, and important reactions versus components that merely interfere or confuse the nervous system—that is, how to avoid false positives and false negatives.

People who have worked with me, especially if it was more than six years ago, may have achieved variable results if we didn't address the components most relevant to their condition. Early in practice, all the pieces of the Protocol had not been established. Now if a patient isn't getting a result, we identify what aspect of the Protocol isn't being followed by identifying the associated muscle weaknesses and reflex points, or we determine if the pieces just need more time to work, or I refer them out to screen for disease if they are not responding to care in a predictable manner.

It's frustrating for me and the patient if we work together for six or seven weeks and they are 90 percent compliant but give up before they have a solution. My intention is not to be overly attached to the outcome while being committed to guiding people to a positive result. I tell people their chances of achieving excellent results increase if they carefully follow the Protocol for two months and follow up with me a few times during that process, but when they can't do it and they don't get the results, it often feels to me that a great opportunity was missed for both of us.

This book is dedicated to the possibility of *not missing those opportunities.* I am committed to the success of my patients, and to that end, people need to understand the Protocol for Health and have access to a helpful book that can be shared with those for whom they care. It's challenging to give a brief explanation of this system, how it works, and why it's an important breakthrough in healthcare.

The experiences of my patients seem to fall into a few main categories. There are those who tried without success because of the obstacles I've described. There are those who achieved a great result and are now dedicated followers of the Protocol, and there are those who achieved a great result but either forgot about it, couldn't maintain it, or didn't realize the full scope of what is possible with this system of healthcare.

Unfortunately, in practice people don't always recognize the significance of a positive outcome. Sometimes I guide a patient to a solution, they succeed where previously they failed, and still they say, "Yeah, it's all better, but I expected fireworks." Holistic healing, which addresses the whole body and affects all systems, often occurs without a patient's awareness. They expect a pop or a magic pill or some weird therapy to be the solution, but we simply remove obstacles to healing. This isn't what people have been conditioned to expect. If they have a relapse or some new symptom, ideally, they recognize that one of the seven factors has drifted out of balance and needs to be identified and addressed, but too often they forget how easily we can do that, or they decide it means the Protocol doesn't work or is too difficult.

While I'm describing this protocol in detail, this isn't a complete how-to book, and it shouldn't be used as a recommendation, treatment, or diagnosis for any condition. I don't specialize in managing disease but in guiding people to health. The Protocol can reverse chronic illness, but serious illness should be managed or co-managed by a medical doctor or disease specialist. In serious situations medical interventions should be available to control symptoms while addressing the underlying conditions that created the illness. Identifying underlying causes with instant, accurate feedback from the body helps us identify and address the seven main causes of disease, but drugs and surgery rarely if ever address an underlying cause. When poor health or an unidentified issue has progressed too far and there is serious disease, powerful emergency intervention of the medical profession may be our only hope, and we are glad that system is available for managing those conditions. However, that's not a system that has much motivation or sensitivity to identify and address the causes of most health conditions.

It's important that people take a more active role in their own healthcare and stop expecting a solution from a doctor, a pill, or a machine, but it's also important to remember there is no substitute for the thousands of hours of training, testing, and continuing education required to be a doctor of any type. Many people have lost faith in their doctors as it becomes clear that most of our systems of healthcare, with the exception of emergency care, don't work very well, and doctors are rarely able to guide patients or themselves in regimens that consistently restore health and resolve symptoms. However, it's still important to safely screen for and rule out serious conditions so that we can work on creating health without overlooking a condition that may not allow us the time we need to address the underlying issues.

I won't claim to treat serious illness or prevent disease with the Protocol until there are studies that confirm its effectiveness *for those purposes*. In the meantime, I offer safe, simple, effective, holistic solutions that consistently resolve symptoms and restore health.

CHAPTERS 4 through 10

Solutions to the Seven Underlying Causes of Disease

CHAPTER 4
The First Cause of Disease and the Unexpected Solution

Pervasive Chronic Intestinal Infection

The Lancet medical journal published a study about zinc and atmospheric CO_2 in 2015 that led me to develop the flow chart on the next page. Researchers showed that as CO_2 increases, plants uptake less zinc and a few other essential minerals. As a result, the meat and vegetables we eat generally contain less zinc than before industrialization. While the study doesn't suggest this factor directly affects most of us living in industrialized nations, a much bigger issue could be hidden by a small error in the estimates for adequate zinc intake and uncertainties about our ability to absorb and utilize it. It is also unknown how much zinc intake has decreased because of dietary changes after the invention of agriculture and because of modern environmental degradation.

There is no accurate laboratory test for zinc deficiency. Estimates for the prevalence of the deficiency vary greatly, and there's minimal agreement among various sources for effective zinc supplementation methods. This is a massive blind spot in our health.

With muscle testing, I find almost all new patients to be deficient in zinc. Addressing this deficiency is an essential piece of resolving and preventing symptoms. Zinc deficiency leads

ZINC DEFICIENCY—INTESTINAL INFECTION FLOWCHART

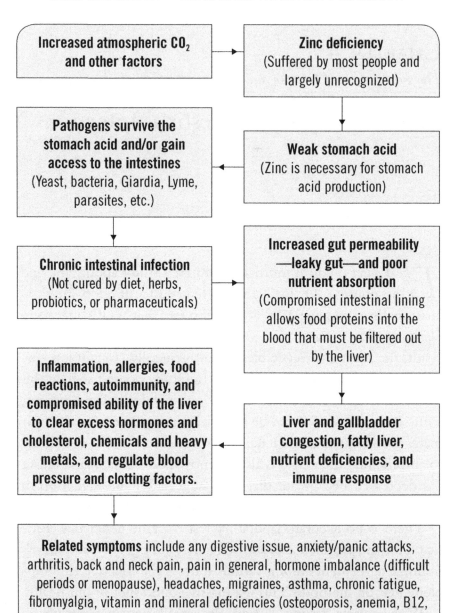

to weak stomach acid, poor absorption, and chronic intestinal infection that contributes to most conditions.

According to the World Health Organization, one-third of the world's population is deficient in zinc. The worst effects are mostly in the developing world—zinc deficiency causes about a million deaths per year, with 193,000 of those due to the deficiency increasing the severity of malaria. The majority of deaths are from pneumonia and diarrhea in children less than five years old. Zinc deficiency is associated with issues of the skin, hair, eyes, mouth sores, wound and tissue healing, loss of senses of vision, smell, and taste, compromised immune function, depression, schizophrenia, complications in pregnancy, poor growth in children, issues with cell division and replication, low testosterone, prostate issues, delayed puberty, inability to mature sexually, and lack of appetite.

While the majority of the most extreme examples of zinc deficiency are reported in the developing world, the deficiency is found in all countries among people with poor diets or poor digestion and is exacerbated by phytates in a plant-based diet. As with all minerals, there is significant uncertainty about optimal intake, blood levels, and the factors that interfere with zinc absorption and utilization. Current research has no consensus on how to test for the deficiency or how to ensure absorption. As with calcium, just because a supplement is absorbed, doesn't mean it functions as intended in the body. Some studies support the use of zinc supplements in the developing world, and sometimes those supplements improve severe health issues, but the results are inconsistent.

The gap between adequate intake of vitamins and minerals to prevent illness or death and *ideal intake for optimal health* is usually difficult or impossible to determine. In modern healthcare we rarely see the full benefits of any vitamin or mineral supplied by foods or supplements because most people either can't fully absorb them, or they can't absorb them in a form that works within the body due to weak stomach acid, zinc deficiency, problematic supplements, and/or dietary complications.

Clear answers through a patient's nervous system can help close this gap and approach optimal intake and absorption. My system of muscle testing demonstrates that almost all new patients are zinc deficient, and that established patients often have recurring obstacles to zinc absorption. Addressing the deficiency is a key to the success of the Protocol for Health, and when combined with clearing chronic intestinal infection, addressing zinc deficiency is a key to addressing most modern health issues.

Zinc deficiency leads to weak stomach acid and compromised immune function, which allows pathogens to survive the stomach acid and create chronic intestinal infection, which may or may not create digestive complaints. Chronic intestinal infection is a catch-all term that includes problematic yeast (Candida), bacteria (small intestinal bacterial overgrowth—SIBO—or other forms), Giardia (protozoa), and parasites. In my practice there is rarely an exact diagnosis of the type of infection, but which type of infection makes little difference for the Protocol: all of these infections can be cleared with a twenty-day course of enzymes. Normally, these types of infections are considered quite difficult to eliminate, and the medical and alternative treatments designed to poison the infection are known to have side effects, such as Herxheimer reaction, bacterial die-off, fatigue, headaches, worsened chronic symptoms, or colon cancer for the drug metronidazole (meh·truh·nai·duh·zowl).

The twenty-day course of enzymes my patients take between meals amplify natural digestion in the intestines to break down the defenses of the pathogen and eliminate the infection. The Protocol resolves laboratory-confirmed Giardia, chronic yeast overgrowth, chronic or post-treatment Lyme disease, some tropical diseases, and various types of worms. Some pathogens that create chronic intestinal infection can be introduced to the blood by mosquito or tick bites, contaminated surgeries, other invasive procedures, through the lungs, or other routes.

Generally, the term dysbiosis, rather than chronic intestinal infection, is used to describe issues with intestinal flora that suggest an imbalance or underrepresentation of beneficial bacteria and/or other components of the gut microbiota. Because I find that almost everyone has the condition, and that it tests easily as either present or absent, and can be resolved with a course of enzymes and prevented from returning when strong stomach acid is maintained, I think the condition is more accurately described as pervasive, chronic intestinal infection. This distinction reflects the effectiveness of working with the body with enzymes to amplify digestion between meals to eliminate an infection rather than perpetually adding various types and ratios of beneficial bacteria in new and unusual ways to try to restore balance to the gut. While the latter approach often shows glimpses of encouraging results, the outcomes of supplementing with or consuming probiotics are variable and inadequate for most significant conditions, but the use of enzymes within the Protocol is consistently effective.

Most chronic intestinal infection in the U.S. is probably associated with food poisoning or travelers' diarrhea, which is caused primarily by poor food handling in restaurants or agriculture. Close contact with family members or a companion may also be the source of infection. Frequently however, from the medical laboratory perspective, no pathogen or cause can be identified with the onset of digestive complaints and diarrhea.

Researching digestive conditions in general, it becomes clear that causes for most intestinal conditions are usually uncertain. Significant overlap in symptoms for travelers' diarrhea, IBS, celiac disease, IBD, colitis, and Crohn's disease makes it difficult to obtain a clear diagnosis. This overlap combined with the vast number of possible pathogens that may be involved, but are frequently unidentified, makes it especially unlikely to receive effective treatment for these conditions. With the confusion around diagnosis, it becomes difficult to track the prevalence of these issues. Most of these conditions are becoming more common, but to what degree is unknown. It's also established that infections that are identified as the cause of symptoms and disease for some can be present in others with no digestive complaints. These facts support my theory that the healthcare system has a limited ability to diagnose and treat pervasive chronic intestinal infection and recognize its contribution to most health and/or digestive issues.

Chronic intestinal infection of all types irritates the intestinal lining, which causes increased permeability and leaky gut, which allows food proteins to be absorbed before they are broken down into smaller amino acids. Food proteins in the blood are treated as foreign invaders by the immune system and cause an immune response every time we eat. This constant immune response to *simply eating* contributes to inflammation, allergies, food allergies, a weak immune system, and likely cancer as well.

Even if one is eating an optimal diet, undigested food proteins in the blood cause inflammation and must be filtered out of the blood by the liver. Constantly filtering large proteins compromises or stresses the liver. This is liver congestion and may also be the driver of fatty liver. The liver passes whatever sludge it can to the gallbladder to be stored until being eliminated through the small intestine. If this overwhelms the gallbladder, stones and/or gallbladder attacks may result. Gallbladder attacks or congestion, which often cause nausea or pain in the upper abdomen or the middle of the back, are easily resolved with the Protocol. Liver and gallbladder congestion compromise our ability to clear chemicals, pharmaceuticals, antibiotics, pesticides, heavy metals, and our own excess hormones and cholesterol, all of which lead to other conditions.

Many in the alternative health field believe that dysbiosis, leaky gut, inflammation, digestive issues, and a variety of other conditions are caused by pesticides, glyphosate, antibiotics, or other synthetic or natural chemicals such as lectins in nightshades. Of course, all of these can become significant irritants, and many people can link their symptoms to exposure to these chemicals. When chronic intestinal infection is cleared and the Protocol is in place, minimal exposure to these irritants no longer triggers serious issues. That said, I certainly think we should avoid pesticides when possible, use antibiotics only when necessary, and recognize that while food sensitivities can be very significant, many food sensitivity reactions can be reduced or eliminated.

Almost all of my established patients can eat conventional, non-organic meat, eggs, and vegetables without symptoms, even if pesticides used to cause them problems. Patients who must take a course of antibiotics for dental work or some other issue may not feel as well while they are taking them. However, they recover without taking probiotics within a couple days of finishing the pharmaceutical, even if they blamed their previous health issues on past antibiotic exposure, and even if they used to benefit from supplementing with probiotics. Patients who previously reacted to nightshades and suffered from mouth sores, arthritis, or other conditions caused by consuming tomatoes or other foods can almost always reintroduce these foods without symptoms. While the entire Protocol is involved in reducing these reactions, clearing intestinal infection is almost certainly the most important piece, as it stops leaky-gut and clears liver congestion.

With a system of objective muscle testing, it's possible to see clear indicators in the form of reflex points and muscle weaknesses for each of the steps in the Zinc Deficiency—Intestinal Infection Flowchart, which are associated with corresponding symptoms. The indicators and symptoms resolve when an effective solution is applied. When conditions are created for clear muscle testing, chronic intestinal infection causes a pattern where a person weakens to two different reflex points. It also causes weakness of the tensor fasciae latae muscles (TFLs)(Figure 4 below) that connect to the iliotibial or IT band, and the psoas major muscles are usually weak as well (Figure 3 page 31). These reflexes clear and the associated muscles temporarily strengthen when a person tastes the enzymes that will clear the intestinal infection, and they stay strong after the enzymes are taken consistently for twenty days to clear the infection.

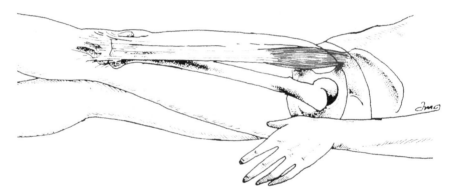

4. Tensor Fascia Lata. From the pelvis to the knee.

While this technique has not been medically established beyond our practice, it is easy to demonstrate, the changes in muscle strength are dramatic—often ten times or more—and the results are consistent and profound. When the psoai and TFLs strengthen, the opposing muscles of the low back can relax, which decreases the likelihood of symptoms of low back or hip pain. At the same time, people who complain of intestinal dysfunction or pain usually resolve these issues as the enzymes start to work. I see patients with long-term low back pain, diarrhea, constipation, and more severe issues quickly heal with this approach. Beyond case studies or miracle stories, the consistency with which related muscles strengthen and associated symptoms clear is most revealing. The Protocol consistently strengthens muscles and clears symptoms.

Ideally, laboratory tests would always be able to identify chronic intestinal infection. While many pathogens can be identified, some are known to be difficult or impossible to determine, and lab work in this arena can be experimental and uncertain. People frequently come to me who have undergone many tests for infection, but nothing was found. I usually confirm the presence of chronic intestinal infection with the pattern of reflexes and muscle weaknesses as described. When I find intestinal infection and utilize the enzyme regimen with patients, we see the pattern of weakness and related symptoms clear. Lab tests look for abnormal findings, usually by comparing results to some supposed, healthy normal average, but if most people have intestinal infection of some form, comparison to normal findings doesn't reveal an abnormal finding. It's normal and essential for thousands of different types of bacteria, yeast, and other microbes to live in the digestive tract. While science is working at determining which are pathogenic versus those that are beneficial, there is a long way to go. The Protocol consistently clears discomfort and dysfunction. Perhaps lab work done before and after the enzyme protocol could determine which pathogens are being cleared and therefore gain insight into their pathogenic nature. While that could be a useful academic study, it's unlikely it would change my method for identifying and clearing chronic intestinal infection.

Perhaps part of the reason that the use of enzymes for clearing intestinal infection is unknown or not practiced is because it can make some patients uncomfortable or will not accomplish the desired result if improperly managed. Chronic intestinal infection causes leaky gut, which causes liver and gallbladder congestion, but taking the enzymes temporarily makes more work for the liver and the gallbladder. The enzymes can cause liver-related symptoms of nausea, headaches, upper back pain, acne, and malaise. It's difficult to predict which patients will experience these symptoms. In general, older patients and those with more advanced conditions need to be managed more carefully, but even people in those groups often feel better while taking the enzymes. Occasionally, even athletes in their twenties need to slow the process to stay reasonably comfortable. In the days and months after the twenty-day enzyme regimen, the full spectrum of people experience improvements in health and a decrease in overall symptoms.

The best methods for supporting the process of taking the enzymes are to eat a good, simple diet (Simple Foods Diet on page 77), include a lot of cooked vegetables if tolerated, drink extra water, and walk as described in Chapter 9. If possible, follow up one to four days after starting the enzymes and once every week or two for the first six to eight weeks of care with myself or another healthcare provider who has an understanding of the Protocol for Health. If people are working with the enzymes on their own, it is particularly important to start slowly and to slow or stop the process with any increase of significant negative symptoms. Usually, giving the body a couple of days to catch up with the process allows the enzymes to be restarted with little or no symptoms. Occasionally, people are unable to proceed without additional help. Cooked vegetables are usually helpful as they are easy for most to digest, and the vegetable fiber helps carry waste products out of the body, decreasing reabsorption of these potentially irritating components. Drinking extra water means drinking one quart per fifty pounds of body weight per day, or more for those who exercise frequently.

Soon after a person starts the enzymes, with follow-up testing we can determine if the liver or gallbladder needs additional support through the process. My testing usually confirms the gallbladder is the next piece to address, which is usually cleared by holding a couple of sets of reflex points (Chapter 11). Holding reflex points doesn't seem like it would create a solution, but it clears muscle weakness, addresses meridian pulse points, and helps with symptoms as it supports the process. Before discovering this technique, I used supplements frequently for liver and gallbladder, but now I use those only with patients with advanced conditions or recent gallbladder issues. Whether or not additional supplements for liver and gallbladder are needed in the process, most patients experience improvements in liver, gallbladder, and intestinal-related symptoms, and certain blood tests improve as well. The process simultaneously clears chronic intestinal infection and the related liver and gallbladder congestion, and patients are usually comfortable in the process.

When new patients come in with gallbladder attacks or other related symptoms, we're able to resolve these problems with the Protocol as long as a patient isn't in an emergency situation. Gradually softening the contents of the gallbladder with a supplement made from beets while taking betaine hydrochloride (HCl) and the twenty days of enzymes allow the gallbladder to gently clear, which in turn enables the liver to more effectively filter waste products from the body. Because of how consistently gallbladder attacks are resolved and the fact that I've never seen an established, adherent patient develop gallbladder issues, I think chronic intestinal infection is the biggest driver of gallbladder issues. Additionally, I have always found the presence of intestinal infection with patients who have previously had their gallbladders removed.

Stressed liver and gallbladder both have two reflex points that weaken a previously strong muscle, and liver congestion creates a predictable weakening of the sternal head of the pectoralis major muscles. This weakness causes opposing tension and possible pain in the upper back and neck and/or tension headaches common in our society. These symptoms usually clear when liver congestion and its cause are addressed. Another symptom of liver congestion is poor hormone regulation, which often presents as difficult menstrual periods or menopause. It's rewarding to work with these complaints because I can virtually guarantee significant improvement within two or three months, if not sooner. The liver clears excess estrogen or estrogen-like chemicals from the body, so clearing liver congestion and its cause dramatically improves hormone elimination, regulation, and balancing. Similar results are achieved for men who appear to be low in testosterone.

The effects of the supplements and diet are illustrated by the predictable reduction of the above symptoms and lasting benefits when people continue to take absorbable zinc and betaine HCl. If symptoms are related to liver, gallbladder, or intestinal issues, they usually resolve with the enzymes combined with a good diet and the rest of the Protocol. This isn't a treatment for cancer, but in time I think it will be established that liver congestion and intestinal infection are some of the biggest predisposing factors for cancer. When the liver is congested with food proteins, we can't effectively clear excess hormones, chemicals, heavy metals, and waste products—some of the known causes of cancer.

Of the seven main causes of pain and disease, addressing chronic intestinal infection is usually the place to start. Most people have it, it contributes to most symptoms, and it interferes with the absorption of nutrients, elimination of waste products, and regulation of hormones. Chronic intestinal infection creates a pattern of muscle weakness that is perhaps the greatest cause of low back pain, mid back pain, and pain or tension in the upper back and neck. Food allergies and sensitivities are also driven by this issue. Chronic intestinal infection can be cleared with access to the right digestive enzymes and possibly additional supplements for the liver and gallbladder. After it's cleared, recurrence can be prevented by maintaining strong stomach acid.

The enzymes I use with most patients are Zymex II from Standard Process. These were developed roughly eighty years ago by Royal Lee, and while he made more significant claims, the company now simply describes Zymex II as a digestive aid. If patients are especially sensitive or there is a chance of an allergy to almonds or figs, which are in Zymex II, I use Enzyme Defense from Enzymedica instead. The benefits of Enzyme Defense, as described by Enzymedica, are said to be related to immune function, circulation, and the breaking down of excess mucus. Both companies either don't know the full capability of these enzymes, or they limit their claims to be compliant with the guidelines of the Food and Drug Administration. With either supplement, the first couple doses should only amount to one capsule or a part of a capsule's contents until a person confirms that there is no increase in diarrhea, nausea, or other negative symptoms. If these negative symptoms initially occur, they usually resolve if people skip a day and try a small dose again. Some people may need to switch to the other enzyme or work with other aspects of the Protocol for a couple of weeks before they can take the enzymes comfortably. Not all forms of digestive enzymes clear chronic intestinal infection. On the few occasions patients brought in other more expensive brands of enzymes to use for clearing intestinal infection, they were ineffective, but there are probably others that could be used.

Most of my patients increase the dose over a few days—up to nine capsules per day of Zymex II or six per day of Enzyme

Defense. In either case, the supplements are split into three doses taken about two hours after a meal, and then they wait at least an hour before eating again. This is maintained for twenty days or until the patient has finished 180 capsules of Zymex II or 120 of Enzyme Defense.

Sometimes it can be challenging to keep people comfortable in the process, but by following the rest of the Protocol and with some follow-up visits, it's usually gentle. While it's important to be fairly consistent in taking the enzymes, with any unreasonable symptoms, it's important to slow or stop the enzymes for one to four days to allow the body to catch up with the process. Sometimes people make the mistake of trying to power through discomfort, and for some that can become unreasonable with headaches, back pain, nausea, intestinal distress, exhaustion, or flaring of a skin condition. These symptoms are avoided with follow-up appointments and slowing the enzymes if need be.

Some people feel better while they are taking the enzymes and some feel worse, but a week after finishing the enzymes, if the other pieces of the Protocol are mostly in place, they feel better and continue to improve for weeks or months afterward.

Some want to repeat the enzymes because of a return of symptoms or an unresolved condition, but if my testing for intestinal infection confirms it has been eliminated, another round of the enzymes won't achieve the desired result. In this situation, testing or conversation usually determines the aspect of the Protocol not in place, and addressing it achieves the desired result.

Early in the development of the Protocol, people's conditions frequently improved for a few weeks, but then symptoms returned. This can occur when implementing any beneficial component, such as removing gluten from the diet, or other pieces that are helpful but aren't the full solution. Now, if patients have a return of symptoms, we can determine the cause and address it.

Giardia, or the infection of giardiasis, also known as Beaver Fever, is a form of intestinal infection that affects 3 to 7 percent of people in the U.S. It's often treated with the drug metronidazole with the rare but possible side effect of colon cancer. To make it worse, there's growing drug resistance in Giardia, and many people are unaware they are carriers for the infection, which allows it to spread with poor hygiene. Giardiasis is known to affect the permeability of the gut lining, which is why it's associated with the development of food allergies, lactose intolerance, and irritable bowel syndrome even after the infection has cleared. It's also known to cause malabsorption of nutrients such as vitamin A, B-12, and folate, and can lead to skin conditions, joint inflammation, chronic fatigue, failure to thrive in infants or poor growth—all of which overlap with the symptoms of non-specific chronic intestinal infection that I identify.

On the positive side, laboratory testing for Giardia is more likely to be accurate than for other forms of intestinal infection, especially with repeated tests, and it always clears with the enzymes. I don't claim to diagnose giardiasis with manual muscle testing or claim to treat it with enzymes that haven't been proven by others to be effective for treating it, but on the occasions when people have come to me with this diagnosis, their symptoms quickly resolved, and those who retested for Giardia with laboratory tests no longer had it. Muscle testing for chronic intestinal infection can only identify the presence or absence of infection, so I have no way of knowing how many people who come to me have Giardia, Candida, SIBO, or any of the multitude of other forms of chronic intestinal infection. Giardiasis provides an excellent opportunity to prove attainable outcomes with enzymes because it's fairly common and can be diagnosed with lab tests. It would make for a revolutionary large-scale study.

While there are a wide variety of diagnoses that people are

given for their intestinal complaints, most symptoms fall on a spectrum of dysfunction. Whether it's IBS, IBD, Crohn's, colitis, diverticulitis, gastroparesis, constipation, chronic diarrhea, or pain, my solution is mostly the same. As long as the diagnosis isn't cancer, the Protocol is very helpful. With extremely sensitive people, the Protocol is sometimes uncomfortable, but most people feel fine or better through the process. Certainly, there are extreme, dangerous, and/or unstable conditions I would not attempt to treat until a patient was stable and was being carefully co-managed with a gastroenterologist. Autoimmune conditions such as colitis, which respond well to the Protocol, require a greater level of caution and patient compliance as they can flare and become life-threatening. As far as the normal spectrum of digestive diseases, we see great results with patients who follow the Protocol.

Many with chronic intestinal infection have no digestive complaints and are unaware they have it or that it's the cause of such symptoms as headaches, shoulder and back pain, hormone imbalance, arthritis, allergies, etcetera. Of course, this can be confusing to patients, but it's well established that people can be carriers of infections like Giardia or problematic bacteria or yeast but have no obvious digestive symptoms. These people still have the pattern of muscle weakness and reflex points associated with intestinal infection that clears with digestive enzymes. Their health is compromised more or less by poor absorption, poor waste product elimination, and increased inflammation. Clearing these obstacles is essential to achieving results with digestive and non-digestive symptoms alike.

Underlying intestinal infection can be especially problematic and confusing for people who had relatively good health until they were in a car accident or other physical or emotional trauma. Injuries may be difficult to heal without addressing the digestive component. Tight upper trapezii muscles caused by intestinal infection complicates the healing of whiplash or other neck and shoulder injuries, but soon after an accident is a challenging time to suggest that a patient address a digestive issue that they are unaware of and can't connect to their symptoms or healing process. However, addressing digestion at this time can make the difference between an injury that heals in a reasonable amount of time or an injury that leads to chronic pain, disability, pain-medication dependency or an opioid addiction. It's also established that physical or emotional trauma can cause the onset of autoimmunity, digestive problems, or other conditions with poorly understood origins. However, underlying *asymptomatic* chronic intestinal infection could explain many of these mysterious onsets and help people realize that emotional stress is not necessarily the underlying cause of physical symptoms.

While I can't be certain if the overall data are there to quantify it, it seems people have become more prone to chronic injuries and digestive issues of all types, and in general people don't heal as easily as they used to. While the rapid increase of the prevalence of chronic low back pain is well established, most forms of chronic pain and digestive issues aren't tracked as carefully. Changes in the field of chiropractic illustrate recognition of decreasing effectiveness of manual therapies when not combined with a more holistic approach. There is a growing trend for doctors of all types to incorporate systems for addressing digestion and overall health. Some chiropractors complain that it used to be much easier to help patients resolve their injuries and pain, and it seems adjustments used to be more effective at relieving symptoms. It has become more difficult to achieve lasting results. If the prevalence of chronic intestinal infection has rapidly increased in the past few decades, then so has chronic weakness of the associated muscles, as well as the issues of poor absorption, poor elimination, and excessive inflammation. Manual therapies such as chiropractic, physical therapy, and deep tissue massage are less likely to be effective with the presence of chronic intestinal infection because of the obstacles to healing it creates.

Of the seven main causes of disease, it is pervasive chronic intestinal infection that most strongly accounts for the trend of increasing health issues. Increased injuries in all levels of sports are being documented with varying explanations. Repetitive stress injuries and microtrauma from sports or even mild activities are blamed for creating debilitating symptoms. Serious digestive complaints are more common and being reported in younger patients. Much of the opioid epidemic is a reflection of the overall inability to effectively heal and address musculoskeletal injuries and the chronic pain which results. While more professionals and researchers recognize that many or most conditions originate in the gut, the solution and the scope have not been realized. Accurate, instantaneous feedback from the body reveals the pervasive nature of chronic intestinal infection, enables prevention of its return, and guides the course of related factors for achieving the resolution of symptoms.

Many alternative health practitioners attempt to treat various forms of chronic intestinal infection with Candida diets, enemas, or natural forms of poison such as black walnut, cayenne, wormwood, or concentrated oregano, or their goal is often to build up beneficial intestinal flora so that it can restore balance to the gut. While these remedies may help to varying degrees or make the person worse, I haven't seen these treatments remove indicators for chronic intestinal infection.

Whether or not a person experiences benefits from probiotics, fermented foods, L-glutamine, aloe vera, colostrum, and the like, all become unnecessary once intestinal infection is cleared. I used to recommend probiotics and L-glutamine for my patients, but now I almost never do. Beneficial bacteria already live in the gut. It's a symbiotic relationship. If you have to continually add probiotics to feel better, it's because something in the gut keeps killing them off or is more successful in that environment. Once intestinal infection is cleared, beneficial bacteria bounce back naturally, and adding probiotics or fermented foods become optional or unnecessary. Again, while symptoms can sometimes be reduced by probiotics or fermented foods, studies show that for the general population, they work only slightly better than a placebo.

Medical treatments and antibiotics for intestinal infection can be lifesaving, but for a non-lethal infection or chronic intestinal infection, safer options should be considered first. Known side effects for one of the most commonly used drugs of this type, metronidazole, include seizures, meningitis, nerve damage, bad interactions with alcohol, yeast overgrowth, and colon cancer. While some of those side effects may be rare, using this drug for a non-life-threatening condition seems reckless. Then again, when desperate for a solution and the benefits are emphasized and the side-effects are downplayed, it can seem a reasonable choice. But these types of drugs may exacerbate the problem or create other serious health issues. While there are safer forms of antibiotics that eliminate certain infections and may or may not improve symptoms, I've never been able to confirm with my testing that they clear the chronic intestinal infection that most people have. I don't treat conditions that are immediately life-threatening, but chronic stable issues or less severe acute conditions can be treated with this method without risk of significant side effects, and the solution contributes to overall health. My testing shows the presence or absence of intestinal infection, so while an antibiotic may clear findings from lab tests, there are pervasive forms of chronic intestinal infection that often remain unidentified with lab work.

Once intestinal infection is cleared, taking an absorbable zinc supplement with betaine hydrochloride (HCl) helps the body maintain strong stomach acid so a new infection is unlikely to gain access to the intestines. Unfortunately, this means taking a zinc supplement forever, or until we can absorb it more effectively from the diet, but it's rare that patients who stay consistent with quality zinc and HCl return to my office with intestinal infection. I commonly see a patient a few times and we resolve most or all of their symptoms, but despite my recommendation for occasional checkups, I don't see them for a year or two or more. Then they come back to say their symptoms returned. Often in this case, they stopped the zinc or HCl, switched to some other brand, or perhaps just failed to increase the HCl in a period of high stress, poor diet, or cold or flu. We then clear intestinal infection again, and I remind them of the importance of the supplements.

I could try to make a list of all the symptoms connected to intestinal infection (part of that list is at the bottom of my flowchart shown previously), but it's hard to know what to leave off. For example, I've worked with people with heart disease who could barely walk up their driveway but were fine within a month of starting care. Did we clear heart disease? I don't know, but they were able to return to an active lifestyle. I've had great success with narcolepsy, digestive system paralysis (gastroparesis), low milk production in nursing mothers, and chronic or post-treatment Lyme disease, to name a few unusual or difficult cases. The treatment is fundamentally the same as for most low back pain, headaches, arthritis, and digestive complaints—a few basic issues, with chronic intestinal infection as a foundation, underlie most pain and disease.

Here is an example of a typical route to acquiring intestinal infection. Near the end of writing this book I was helping my neighbor with some fire-hazard brush removal. She refilled a couple of water bottles for me while I was working. After almost drinking a half-gallon, I remarked on the good taste of the water.

She told me that she didn't trust her well water and that this water had come from Bitney Springs.

Bitney Springs is a roadside "spring" near our home. The spring has been improved so that water is constantly flowing out of a pipe, and during most daylight hours, people are there filling water bottles or large containers. While there is a nice little permanent shade structure and other improvements there, there now is also a substantial sign that says, "Drink at your own risk," and "Not monitored or tested by (the) county." The county used to test the water but because it always failed and came back positive for coliform bacteria, they would post signs, and then people would tear the signs down. The presence of coliform doesn't necessarily mean the water will cause infection. In this case, the water tastes great, there are stories of healing properties, and it almost certainly was the source of a new case of intestinal infection for me. I have previously made a point of avoiding this water.

About ten days after drinking the water, I found myself in a moment of reflection. I was having an altered and sub-par bathroom experience. As I considered the previous few days, I recalled my poor mood, being unusually tired the day after hard work, and some atypical low back pain. Ten days is a normal incubation period for an ingested pathogen. I guided my wife in muscle testing me and we confirmed intestinal infection.

Without knowing what I know and having this kind of system of testing, it is unlikely I would have connected the dots or been able to easily clear this condition. Would my body have eventually cleared it without intervention? Would I have even noticed a new infection if I already had intestinal infection? Would I have just made a truce with the infection and become a carrier for it? Would there have been some eventual perceived health benefit? (Some studies do suggest intentionally adding certain types of intestinal infection for some perceived benefits—I think that is a bad idea.) Or would it have led to the onset of a variety of chronic conditions and a significant decline in my health? I think all of these outcomes are possible depending on the individual and the timing.

There are many ways to introduce intestinal infection into the body. Similar stories to my experience originate from backpacking trips, swimming in rivers, water skiing, international travel, contaminated well water, breeches in city water systems, or just a meal at a local restaurant. If our stomach acid is strong enough and the exposure is small enough, we dodge the infection. Unfortunately, weak stomach acid and intestinal infection are now pervasive, but this solution has the potential to restore health, happiness, and quality of life. The solution may simply clear common annoying conditions, such as acne, bad breath or body odor, constant burping, frequent or foul gas, thinning hair, lethargy, poor mood, mild headaches, or neck pain. All of these mild conditions may point to a larger issue that may eventually cause more serious symptoms.

CHAPTER 5
The Second Cause of Disease and the Unexpected Solution

Food Reactions: Allergies and Sensitivities

The second main cause of pain and disease is the consumption of foods we weren't designed to eat. Most people with health conditions have inflammation and other negative symptoms from consuming corn, soy, gluten, and/or cow dairy but are unable to connect these foods to their symptoms because of continual exposure, chronic intestinal infection, and the rest of the seven causes of disease that complicate the condition. These foods cause specific patterns of muscle weakness and pain as well as general symptoms of inflammation, digestive disturbance, eczema, or other issues. In practice, it's possible to test a patient directly to each of these foods to identify a negative reaction. These foods didn't significantly enter the human diet until we invented agriculture, which doesn't seem to have been long enough for people to adapt to eating them constantly without suffering consequences. They make up the bulk of many dishes, and they're the cheap, subsidized foundations of most prepared foods and food additives.

It's sensible that clearing intestinal infection and eliminating inflammatory foods heals the gut, reduces food reactions in general, and contributes to overall health. These factors cause leaky gut and allow food proteins to be absorbed into the blood where they are treated as foreign invaders and trigger an immune response, even to foods we should be able to eat. When intestinal infection and problematic foods are removed from the diet, the body can absorb nutrients and eliminate waste products more effectively, inflammation decreases, and the gut lining heals. When the gut lining heals and leaky gut stops, most sensitivities and allergies are reduced or eliminated.

This interaction between chronic intestinal infection and eating food irritants drives inflammation in the digestive tract and throughout the body. It's well known that inflammation is the major problem of healthcare, but when do we hear of a solution that actually works? Inflammation inside arteries creates conditions for plaque to accumulate, which causes heart disease and strokes. Arthritis means inflammation in a joint. What causes the inflammation? Colitis is an inflamed colon. Dermatitis. Tendonitis. Bursitis. Inflammatory pain. What condition isn't made worse or simply caused by inflammation? What are the current supposed solutions? Steroids and nonsteroidal anti-inflammatories (NSAIDs), both of which kill tens of thousands of people every year in the U.S. Turmeric is also used with no significant side effects, and while it can be helpful for some, its overall effect is minimal. When you address the causes of inflammation in the body, it's completely obvious. Pain goes away and problems clear up.

A dramatic example of this reduction of inflammation is seen in acute injuries. When people sprain an ankle or tear a tendon or muscle, there's usually significant swelling. Treatment of acute injuries involves managing or attempting to reduce inflammation. Why would the body create an inflammatory response that needs to be externally managed? The excessive inflammatory response is a result of food reactions, intestinal infection, and the other components we address in practice.

I worked with a runner who had frequent sprained ankles that swelled to the size of a football. Not long into care he found his ankles were stronger, but when he did twist one, the inflammation was dramatically less than before. I also had a patient who was doing well in care, but then she completely tore the ACL in her knee in a ski accident. She saw three orthopedic surgeons who couldn't understand why there was almost no inflammation with her torn ACL. Less inflammation means less pain and better healing, whether it's a sprained ankle, herniated disc, "repetitive microtrauma," or gallbladder surgery.

How about the injury that never heals? I broke my wrist about twenty years ago, but seven years later, it was still sensitive and painful with a limited range of motion. The last piece I put in place was to remove gluten from my diet. Two months later, the wrist was 95 percent improved. I avoided gluten for a couple more months and then drank a dark European beer (containing gluten), and my wrist hurt for a couple of days. Again, I avoided gluten for two months until I accidentally ate gluten at a potluck, and my wrist hurt again for a couple of days. Now, more than ten years later, if I eat gluten, which I do occasionally, it doesn't affect the wrist, and even demanding activities don't cause wrist pain. After inflammation was reduced for several months, the wrist finally healed. *That's not normal.* Normal is that old injuries that haven't healed, don't heal, and arthritis progresses until there is disability, surgery, drugs, or a combination of all three. By clearing the causes of inflammation and improving the absorption of needed nutrients, old injuries can heal.

It's typical in my practice that somewhere between a few days to two months into care, patients see improvements in a variety of seemingly unconnected symptoms. Most common are issues like back, neck, or other pain, headaches, digestive issues, low energy, poor sleep, menstrual cramps, leg cramps, and/or allergies. During this time patients may eat one or more of the foods I've suggested they avoid, and as a result they see a setback in their progress. In this manner people prove to themselves, and confirm for me, that even small amounts of offending foods can cause significant symptoms. These are usually people who previously had no idea they were reacting negatively to specific foods, but then they start to pay close attention to the foods they eat. Skeptics like myself suddenly realize that eating a particular food causes significant symptoms and that most of us constantly eat foods that make us sick and cause pain or slowly set us up for the usual train wreck of health decline.

Corn, soy, gluten, and cow dairy—the four common food irritants—are everywhere in our diets and other products, and even small amounts often cause significant and specific symptoms. If people eat these foods frequently, they most likely don't notice that very small amounts may affect how they feel. For example, it may not make sense to eliminate spaghetti sauce in a jar that contains citric acid made from GMO corn, until a patient stops eating corn chips and popcorn. To observe a change in symptoms from eliminating food irritants from the diet, people may need to clear intestinal infection and strengthen stomach acid before and/or during the process of carefully eliminating these possible offending foods. The symptoms may be easier to identify if a patient can eliminate all four foods at the same time and eat limited quantities of carbohydrates and adequate protein, but for some patients, this is asking too much. Maybe they can eliminate one food at a time. While this may decrease the chance of obtaining a clear result, I do my best to meet people where they're at. The relationship most of us have with our diets is complicated—emotionally, mentally, physically, and sometimes spiritually.

Several years ago, a patient came to me who was visiting from India. By testing her directly to cow dairy, I determined she was reacting to milk proteins, and I suggested that dairy products might be the cause of her headaches. When she tasted powdered milk her psoas muscles weakened dramatically, and I demonstrated a connection between her weak psoai and tension in the muscles at the base of the back of her head (sub-occipital and/or upper trapezii muscles). She said, "Oh no, doctor. I cannot eliminate dairy from my diet. I am a vegetarian, and this is my main source of protein." I did my best to be unattached to the outcome while I explained the likely connection between her headaches and her diet and suggested other non-meat protein sources. When we had a follow-up appointment about a year later, she said it had taken a few months before she was willing to change her diet, but she found that eliminating cow dairy products eliminated the daily headaches that had affected her for forty years.

These connections between diet and symptoms are far more common than people realize, and unfortunately, moderation isn't the key. The key is recognizing that most people frequently eat foods they weren't designed to eat and to which they have negative reactions that contribute to the healthcare train wreck we are all involved in. This is one of the main causes of constant inflammation, muscle weakness, pain, and hormone issues that are likely to affect everyone sooner or later. Many dieticians and other practitioners take the stance with their clients that there are no bad foods, and people shouldn't feel bad about eating anything. I agree there's no benefit to feeling guilty about food choices, but people need to know if their food is causing symptoms so they can make educated choices and be in control of their health. Until practitioners can accurately identify food allergies and sensitivities, they're limited in their ability to guide their clients to see the effects of the diet for themselves.

Once the main sources of the common food irritants have been eliminated from the diet, people start to make connections between small exposures (or large indulgences) to these foods and specific symptoms. Some random examples are carpal-tunnel-like symptoms from the soy lecithin in a chocolate bar, depressed thyroid or slowed metabolism from soy-based synthetic vitamin E in skin lotion, depression or foggy head from corn-based xanthan gum in gluten-free products, or TMJ dysfunction from corn-based ascorbic acid (synthetic vitamin C) in multivitamins. Cow dairy products often cause low back pain, upper neck pain, and/or headaches. All four foods, whether organic, raw, fermented, or GMO can cause digestive issues, inflammation, and a variety of other general and/or specific symptoms. Virtually everyone who has significant symptoms of any type and then clears intestinal infection and eliminates these foods from the diet is able to confirm that even small amounts of these foods create negative symptoms.

Fortunately, sensitivity to these foods can be decreased, especially after clearing chronic intestinal infection, which eventually enables most people to enjoy them occasionally without significant symptoms. After about six months of avoiding the common food irritants and strengthening the body overall by following the Protocol, most people see a reduction in their reactivity to these foods as well as other irritants like dust, pollen, mold, perfume, bug bites, poison oak, and pathogen-related symptoms, such as colds and flu and recurring infections. Reintroduction of too much of the food irritants usually causes a return of some symptoms that disappear again when the person reduces or eliminates the offending foods again.

While gluten and cow's milk products have received the most attention in healthcare and allergy awareness, my established patients who have reduced their sensitivity to all four irritants usually find that corn and soy continue to be the most problematic, even in small quantities. This is a challenge because most packaged and prepared foods, supplements, multivitamins, and personal care products contain one or both of these foods, often in their worst, most processed forms. While eliminating corn and soy from the diet may be difficult, it creates seemingly miraculous changes with many conditions, especially or sometimes only when combined with clearing chronic intestinal infection. Because corn and soy particularly affect the pituitary and thyroid respectively, these foods are usually involved in glandular and hormonal issues I describe later.

One would think if so many people suffer serious symptoms from common foods, then surely laboratory food allergy or food sensitivity testing could illuminate the issue. The problem is that food allergy and food sensitivity testing haven't been proven to be accurate. All forms of testing are known to yield false positives and false negatives. The gold standard or best test of modern medicine for food allergy and sensitivity is a "food challenge." A food challenge just means that a person avoids a particular food for some time and then, under medical supervision, eats a significant quantity of that food to see how sick they get. While this method doesn't seem especially sophisticated, it's still considered the best food reaction test of modern medicine. Unfortunately, when chronic intestinal infection is present, which is true for most people, even this test is likely to be unclear. For many people the presence of intestinal infection creates a constant baseline of symptoms and secondary sensitivities to foods that aren't truly the primary cause of their issues. In this situation, laboratory testing, or the patient's experience, may suggest they react to dozens of foods or even most foods. Also, testing can be compromised by the fact that corn and soy are ubiquitous. While they may not register negatively on a test, they can be the underlying drivers of reactions to other foods. For these reasons, the most efficient route forward in practice is usually to eliminate all four common food irritants for the first two months of care—easier said than done, but usually worth the effort.

Perhaps the biggest problem with laboratory testing is that test results generally have to be compared to a theoretical, healthy normal average. Unfortunately, what's normal, or accepted, in this country is that sooner or later people develop chronic illness, pain, and disease. *The premature health-decline most people experience is partially driven by constant reactions to common foods.* If an accurate laboratory test is developed but shows that almost everyone reacts to corn, dairy, soy, and wheat—the top four subsidized foods in the U.S—it seems unlikely the results would be accepted.

Further complications and confusion about test results come from the categorization of food allergy, intolerance, sensitivity, and hypersensitivity. A food allergy can be mild to immediately life-threatening, while the other three conditions, which are all basically the same, cause an overall reduction in quality of life and perhaps eventually quantity of life.

With laboratory tests, it's difficult or impossible to differentiate which food allergies and sensitivities are primary, and therefore their symptoms can be reduced but not eliminated, versus those which are peripheral or secondary and can eventually be consumed without negative impact. The Protocol helps people get clear answers and avoid much of the confusion of secondary sensitivities. While eliminating foods that are secondary sensitivities may help a person feel better in the short-term, it doesn't get to the cause of why that food became an irritant, and it may be an unnecessary permanent dietary restriction. For example, reaction to eggs is usually a secondary sensitivity that can be resolved if it's not life-threatening. By addressing primary issues, most sensitivities to eggs resolve.

Reactions to the four main subsidized foods in this country is usually a primary issue. We can usually lessen those sensitivities, but I don't see those reactions completely go away. Perhaps there is a solution to reactions to the four common irritants other than avoidance, but I haven't found it. I don't think we were designed to eat those foods.

Reactions to meat, eggs, vegetables (including nightshades and lectins), and fruit are almost always secondary. Reactions to these foods usually resolve within one to six months of starting the Protocol, but the high-carb forms of these foods are still best consumed in moderation. Reactions to nuts and shellfish can be more difficult, but as long as they're not life-threatening, they can usually be cleared as well.

With my system of manual muscle testing, it's possible to test a person directly to a food or supplement to determine a negative reaction. As with all of my testing, we first establish a clear baseline by finding a strong muscle and confirming that it weakens when the patient touches the reflex point between their eyebrows, confirming they weaken when they should weaken. Then the patient tastes the food in question, and without touching the reflex point, we retest the muscle to see if it weakens. If it weakens, that's a food reaction. If it remains strong, the patient touches the reflex point and we retest to see if the muscle no longer weakens when it should. Either change in testing suggests the food should be avoided at least for the short-term and possibly long-term.

No one has proven that tasting a food or supplement can cause instantaneous and consistent changes in muscle strength that can be used to accurately identify food reactions, so this can't be called a diagnosis as of yet, and I understand skepticism of this technique of testing. However, patients consistently confirm the answers for themselves by eliminating the food from their diet and observing the resolution of symptoms or the return of symptoms when they reintroduce the food, which essentially is a food challenge—the gold standard of medical food allergy testing.

One of the greatest strengths of my technique is using muscle testing to identify issues that lab tests can't. For instance, corn, dairy, and soy each create specific patterns of muscle weakness. If someone has eaten one of these foods in the few days before an office visit, it's usually apparent and can be demonstrated to the patient. In the course of a normal visit, we might identify a person's sensitivity to cow dairy products and that they have eaten some within the past four or five days. We can demonstrate the pattern of muscle weakness dairy has caused and the reflex point at the back of the skull that clears the weakness. This can be powerful feedback as it shows a patient the sensitivity and accuracy of the testing and that even small amounts of problematic foods create obvious weakness. This discovery may help them realize they're consuming a food irritant when they thought they weren't—maybe they didn't realize there was soy in soy sauce or that whey protein is a dairy product or some similar oversight. Keeping a food journal helps to avoid some of these mistakes.

The Paleo diet—or trying to approximate what we ate before the advent of agriculture—is a good general guideline. This means eating simple, whole foods while avoiding the four common food irritants and food additives and significantly reducing intake of carbohydrates, whether fruit, potatoes, grains, legumes, or sugar of any form. The best foods to eat are meat, eggs, vegetables, some nuts, limited amounts of the best forms of carbohydrates like fruit, sweet potatoes, goat yogurt, and small amounts of our favorite decadent desserts. I find most people can include goat and water buffalo dairy products in a Paleo diet without negative impact. These don't contain alpha S1 casein, the protein in cow's milk to which many people react.

When patients start the Protocol, I suggest they eliminate the four food irritants, even though not everyone reacts to all of these foods. Young people without negative symptoms often test fine to some or all of them, but as people get older, and for those dealing with more significant symptoms, it becomes more likely that all four foods are irritants. A good example is a patient of mine who tested fine to dairy products for years, but at some point, in his thirties, he came in with new complaints of excess mucus and low back pain. Retesting confirmed a reaction to cow dairy. While dairy never bothered him in the past, it now causes symptoms including low back pain. Developments like this and the overall prevalence of reactions to these four foods leads me to believe that most people (with an adequate food supply) are healthier without these foods.

Extreme food allergies like those to nuts and shellfish, which can cause life-threatening closure of the airway, or anaphylaxis, seem to be driven by chronic intestinal infection (leaky gut) combined with eating corn, cow dairy, soy, and gluten. While I have seen the reduction of hypersensitivities to nuts, shellfish, and other foods, I don't claim they can always be resolved. Obviously, these conditions have to be managed with great care, and considering the dangers involved, who wants to retest a potentially life-threatening food? An accurate laboratory test would be very helpful here, but unfortunately, none are known to exist. Still, I can safely work with these people to reduce overall inflammation and decrease lesser reactions to other foods, and this means they're less likely to have a severe reaction if accidentally exposed to an allergen. Additionally, these severe allergies often get worse over time, or other foods start to cause serious reactions. This protocol certainly helps easily managed sensitivities, but to know about severe allergies, studies are needed.

It can be difficult to eliminate irritants from the diet, or possibly cosmetics or supplements, and some have to be more careful than others to achieve results. Unaddressed factors (blood sugar instability, deficiencies of nutrients, lack of beneficial exercise, and overconsumption of carbohydrates) may prevent or delay improvement. This can be a difficult point in the process, and if it continues too long, people may tire of waiting for results and drop out of care. Generally, the Protocol works quickly, but if the food irritants aren't eliminated, blood sugar isn't managed, or key deficiencies are unaddressed, complaints may be prolonged, or benefits may not be realized.

Sometimes people notice that if grains or dairy products are organic, fermented, or raw, they don't cause the same symptoms. Some suggest pesticides or genetic modification drive negative reactions. While these factors probably accelerate sensitivity in the population, the problems with the four common food irritants are bigger and older than chemicals and modern processing. Patients test okay to non-organic meat, eggs, or vegetables, and I rarely see these foods cause symptoms with my established patients. In testing, I see no difference when testing ancient grains, raw, organic, A2 dairy products, or fermented forms of food irritants. They all test poorly even though some of these create fewer symptoms for some people, and symptoms develop even with the best forms of these foods. When we choose to eat a food irritant, it should be the healthiest form, but for optimal health, we should eat none of it.

Cancer, diabetes, and unexplained illness including neurologic or mental health issues have been too common for thousands of years. Some in the Paleo diet community connect an increase in disease to the advent of agriculture. Physical anthropologists examining ancient human skeletons quickly determine if they lived before or after the invention of agriculture. Presumably, eating excessive grains and potatoes and settling down to grow crops results in smaller, thinner, less symmetrical skeletons with more signs of disease.

I recommend the following Simple Foods Diet for most new patients on the first visit. Of course, this diet may not fit everyone, but in general these guidelines work well while implementing the rest of the Protocol. For some, this diet is too strict, while others may be unable to eat many of these foods without experiencing symptoms. Those following the full Protocol do well on this diet sooner or later. For my patients who initially have sensitivities to some of these foods (eggs, nuts, goat dairy, certain vegetables), I recommend they continue to avoid those foods for a few weeks or months. They can usually reintroduce these foods eventually without issue. Those who thought they could never cut out sugar and carbs, or eat red meat, or stop eating bread and pasta, usually find the Protocol helps them make those changes, and they experience clear benefits as a result. Some aspects of the Simple Foods Diet are described further in following chapters.

SIMPLE FOODS DIET

A variation of a low-carb Paleo or ketogenic diet. An approximation of the pre-agriculture diet.

Foods to Eat:
- Meat, eggs, and vegetables. Meat should be mostly nitrite/nitrate-free, additive-free, or better quality. While grass-fed and organic products are ideal, for those on a tight budget, conventional meats and vegetables are better than grains as far as personal health is concerned. The other pieces of the Protocol improve the body's ability to eliminate added hormones and pesticides.

- Nuts and seeds in moderation and only if there is no intestinal irritation or diarrhea. Safest to avoid peanuts because of mold and other factors.
- Nut butters in moderation—almond, cashew, sunflower, etc. (not peanut).
- When reducing carbohydrates, you will probably need to increase fat consumption for energy production. You may need to eat more of these foods: butter, avocados, olives, coconut, soy-free mayonnaise, fatty meats, and oils. Cheap oils often include problematic chemical solvents.
- Goat cheese, water buffalo cheese. Goat milk or goat yogurt are okay but are higher in sugars than cheese.
- Coconut milk (canned). Coconut milk in a carton usually contains too many additives.
- Vegetable juice and sauce (carrot, tomato, etc.). Watch out for citric acid and ascorbic acid (usually made from corn).
- Sea salt, spices, mustard, and types of vinegar that are free of additives, MSG, and white vinegar (usually made from corn).
- Possibly organic unsweetened almond or other nut milk. Cheap products often contain chemical solvents, corn, or soy. Those with especially compromised health may need to avoid nuts.

Optional:

- Caffeine in moderation and only within one hour after eating protein. If you drink decaffeinated coffee or tea, it should be "water process" and/or organic and treated as caffeine.
- Wine, but even organic sulfite-free wine usually contains

added corn or chemicals. It's difficult but possible to find wine without problematic additives.

- Distilled spirits (tequila, Scotch and Irish Whiskey, and some brands of vodka test okay) in moderation and best after protein.

Keep Carbohydrates to a Minimum. Avoid most sugar and starch. If you exercise a lot or if your energy crashes with fewer carbs, you may need to add some **reasonable carbs** when starting this diet, such as half a sweet potato, some goat yogurt, or a little fruit. If it's difficult at first, understand it gets easier with the rest of the Protocol in place. Once your condition has stabilized and/or you're about two months into the Protocol, you might experiment with the reintroduction of more carbs, but most people find they feel better with minimal carbs.

Intestines: If you have diarrhea or intestinal discomfort, don't eat spicy foods, raw vegetables, salads, nuts, or seeds (unless ground smooth, maybe), or berries with seeds, and peel any fruit. When the intestines resolve, some of these foods can be reintroduced.

Foods to Avoid:

- Corn, cow dairy, soy, and gluten (wheat, spelt, barley, and rye); ideally, not even in small amounts.
- Grains and pseudo-cereal grains, such as quinoa, amaranth, and buckwheat. Bread, pasta, crackers, oatmeal, cookies, tortillas, chips, and other foods made from grain.
- High-carb, gluten-free products made from rice or other carbs and xanthan gum (usually made from corn).

- Sweets or products made with sweeteners except for possibly stevia. NOW brand powdered stevia tastes better than most stevia and it tests fine.
- Fruit, fruit juice, and dried fruit, but small amounts may be used for flavoring or as described above in carbs.
- Rice, legumes (beans, lentils, and peas), potatoes, and sweet potatoes, but small amounts might be okay.
- Non-organic milk substitutes with sugar, allergens, or solvents (soy, rice, almond, oat, hemp, etc.).
- Highly processed meats, energy/protein bars or drinks, but they might be okay if low carb and additive/allergen-free.
- Sweet soda, beer, energy drinks, sweet wine, bourbon, gin, and sweet alcohol (rum, liqueurs, etc.).
- Flax, blue-green algae, chlorella, spirulina, wheatgrass, reishi mushrooms, and powerful herbs such as ashwagandha, wormwood, valerian, etc.

Eat plenty and often to control cravings. Eat breakfast within thirty minutes of rising. Don't go more than three hours in the busy part of the day without eating protein. You might need to set a timer. After a few weeks, you might try reintroducing a single serving size portion of **reasonable carbs** (see above) at every other meal or less.

When you eat carbs, you will crave more for a day or two. If you eat more carbs during that time, your craving may get out of control. Eating excessive carbs makes a low-carb diet suddenly boring and unappealing.

Mild aerobic exercise increases tolerance and decreases cravings for carbs.

Learn to cook. Look online or for Paleo/keto cookbooks, recipes, and mail-order food or prepared meals. Cooking on a BBQ is easy—no clean-up. Get help from friends, family, support groups, and online blogs.

Try this for two months. Treat it as an experiment, be creative, and feel better!

Cow's Milk Dairy Products

Many people react to cow's milk and are unaware of the negative symptoms it creates. The most common complaints are diarrhea or other digestive upset and for some excess mucus or sinus congestion. Some notice that if lactose is removed or broken down with lactase enzyme supplements or dairy products containing lactase are consumed, digestive complaints improve or disappear. Unfortunately, reaction to dairy goes beyond digestion. Those with lactose intolerance also react to the proteins in milk. Alpha S1 casein, the large protein in cow's milk, which isn't found in human or goat's milk, is probably the worst offender, but people often react to whey protein as well. Reaction to milk proteins causes muscle weakness and/or inflammation whether or not lactose is present. Often in the course of eliminating cow dairy from the diet, people see the improvement of other symptoms beyond digestion, such as headaches, back pain, sinus infections, eczema, seasonal allergies, acne, arthritis, and occasionally various mental health conditions. Using lactase enzymes to circumvent symptoms caused by cow's milk enables the consumption of a food that drives deeper symptoms rarely associated with milk consumption. The same is true for those who eat hard cheese or cow's milk yogurt to avoid symptoms. If people with this sensitivity continue to eat much of these foods, they eventually cause significant symptoms.

Most people who believe they're lactose intolerant can eat goat dairy products without negative symptoms, which is surprising because goat's milk contains nearly as much lactose as cow's milk. While this contradiction is now recognized by some mainstream medical groups, for many years it wasn't. Some medical experts are still adamant that genetically determined insufficiency of enzymes for the digestion of lactose is the problem and that milk proteins are only an issue in rare true allergies. That argument is now receding, and people recognize negative reactions to proteins are on a spectrum of sensitivity. Low-grade constant reactions to common foods are more difficult to diagnose, but they contribute to inflammation, physical stress, and inflammatory pain and therefore chronic illness and most health conditions.

Chronic disease is the biggest issue of modern health, and the treatments of modern medicine aren't very effective. Often, the process is to wait and monitor the indicators until an issue is bad enough to use drugs or surgery to suppress symptoms while failing to address the causes of the issue. General symptoms such as aches, pains, eczema, and inflammation are considered normal because most have them, and there are no established means of identifying the causes or solutions. Laboratory work fails to identify causative issues like negative food reactions, so the collective experts look at lactose intolerance and similar issues and work on ways to suppress the symptoms of eating foods we weren't designed to eat. Until laboratory testing makes significant advances, that system will continue to provide false information.

Testing needs to be specific to an individual, not a comparison to normal test values. It should incorporate the body as a whole. This may only be possible through the nervous system, which is far more powerful than any machine when it comes to information about, and healing of, the body. Clear answers through the nervous system go way beyond what is possible with lab work. When a patient comes to me and we use their body and nervous system to identify muscle weakness and the associated reflex points, we address causative issues. Overall health improves, muscle weakness clears, and "normal aches and pains" resolve. We don't "wait and see;" we clear the issue before it develops into the seemingly random, unavoidable, genetically determined disease process.

Eventually, it will be widely recognized that cow's milk protein is one of the main causes of low back pain. For many, dairy products cause a weakening of the psoas major muscles, which causes opposing tension in the low back. This is related to the negative impact of dairy products on the kidneys and their association with the psoas major muscles. Because intestinal infection is the other main cause of low back pain, eliminating dairy while clearing intestinal infection routinely relieves acute or chronic low back and hip pain. There are a few other common factors that contribute to low back pain described in Chapter 10.

In 2008, I had a couple of visits with a patient in his twenties who had recurring pain-scale measurements of "ten out of ten" for low back pain that started when he was sixteen. Sometimes it was triggered by wearing a backpack, working out, or physical labor, but simple activities like buttering toast or walking across a parking lot could trigger it as well. We addressed a few aspects of his health and demonstrated his reactions to cow's milk and corn. He's been free of low back pain ever since, unless he gets too casual about his diet. Instead of four to twelve chiropractic visits a year for over ten years, we had three visits, and we were done. The unintended side effects of addressing his low back pain are the resolution of his allergies, mid back pain, and indigestion.

Because eliminating dairy is fairly simple and is one of the most important interventions for clearing low back pain, I conducted a study in 2011 to demonstrate this connection. For the study I asked twenty-eight people (not patients of mine) who had low back pain for more than six months to eliminate cow dairy products from their diet with no other new therapies. Over the course of eight weeks they repeatedly scored their symptoms on questionnaires for low back pain disability. At the end of eight weeks, half the study participants averaged a 70-percent improvement in their low back pain scores. In following up with them after the study, I found many of the participants chose to continue to avoid dairy products and as a result had significant continued improvement in their low back pain. The study should have been longer than eight weeks. Also, many of the participants reported improvements in other conditions, such as allergies, digestive disturbance, arthritis, and headaches. If we had cleared intestinal infection at the same time and the study had been lengthened to three or four months, the results would have been even better. Certainly, this was not a large double-blind study, which is nearly impossible to do with diet, but these results could be confirmed with a more robust and longer-lasting study. The study is included in Appendix A.

I give the following to new patients to help them identify and avoid cow dairy products:

Cow Dairy Avoidance

Avoid foods made from cow's milk: milk, cheese, yogurt, sour cream, cream, whipped cream, half and half, cottage cheese, cream cheese, ice cream, whey (milk protein), casein, caseinate, lactalbumin, lactose, and colostrum.

The following foods are likely to contain cow dairy: milk chocolate, custard, pudding, cream soup, sauce, salad dressing, gravy, batter, bread, breaded foods, muffins, cake, cookies, protein drinks, energy bars, candy bars, most desserts, and flavored chips or flavored popcorn.

Problematic dairy alternatives (avoid): soy products (milk, ice cream, cheese, etc.), non-dairy creamer (made with hydrogenated oils and other chemicals), and cow dairy products with added lactase enzyme (still contains milk proteins).

Surprisingly, the following foods sometimes contain cow dairy (check ingredients): margarine, soy cheese, imitation dairy products, non-dairy creamer, salami, lunch meats, sausage, hot dogs, liverwurst, and pâté.

Foods that are not cow dairy (usually okay to eat): eggs, calcium lactate, cocoa butter, cream of tartar, and lactic acid.

Dairy products that are usually okay: most **butter** and ghee (clarified butter) from cow's milk (because the large proteins are removed, except for one brand of popular organic butter which leaves in more of these proteins), and **goat** and **water buffalo** dairy products (even though they contain lactose). Best to avoid sheep dairy products, but they may be okay for some.

Products that are okay for most patients who are cow dairy sensitive (Some of these are high sugar but could work as an occasional treat. Check ingredient labels and watch out for added chemicals or other possible food allergens/irritants): goat milk products such as goat milk, goat yogurt, various goat cheeses (jack, cheddar, gouda, brie, blue, etc.), condensed goat milk, goat cream cheese, goat ice cream (LaLoo), goat whey protein powder, water buffalo mozzarella, organic alternative milks (almond, hazelnut, hemp, rice, etc., but check

> ingredients), coconut milk (canned not boxed, good in coffee and recipes), dark chocolate bars and chocolate chips (watch out for soy), and coconut milk ice cream (Coconut Bliss).

Gluten (wheat, spelt, barley, and rye)

Awareness of the surprisingly common negative impact of gluten has dramatically increased over the last few years, and more and more people are eliminating it from their diets. Mostly, I see gluten contribute to digestive issues, general inflammation, and allergies. It can prevent healing, cause mental health issues, acne or other skin issues, and cause or contribute to autoimmune conditions. Because it usually increases inflammation, any pain or disease process is worsened by the consumption of gluten for those who react to it.

Known reactions to wheat, or gluten in general, include wheat allergy, non-celiac gluten sensitivity, and celiac disease. The latter two are known to affect any part of the body but are most common in the digestive tract, and celiac disease is considered an autoimmune condition. While celiac disease can be a serious condition, it sometimes has no symptoms. It's estimated that 80 percent of cases remain undiagnosed, and it may take up to twelve years to receive a diagnosis after the onset of symptoms. Estimates of its prevalence range from one in three hundred to one in forty. To conclusively identify celiac disease, a variety of tests are required, including multiple biopsies of tissue from the small intestine. These biopsies are collected with a form of endoscopy that pushes a device down the throat, through the stomach, and into the small intestine. This risky procedure has a complication rate of greater than one in one hundred requiring additional hospitalization. While the only known effective treatment for celiac disease is a gluten-free diet, it's said to be critical to continue to eat gluten until a diagnosis can be determined. This seems like marginal advice because of the requirement of continued exposure to an irritant and the fact that medical testing for celiac disease includes death as a possible complication.

I describe the prevalence of celiac disease, its hidden nature, and the difficulty and danger involved in confirming the diagnosis not to criticize modern medicine but because people should know how common the issue is and how difficult it is to diagnose. I can't distinguish celiac disease from any other form of gluten reaction, but I can identify if a patient reacts to gluten and show them how to reduce the severity of the reaction. This approach is easy, safe, fast, affordable, and accurate.

There are many brilliant discoveries and abilities of modern science and medicine, but simple accurate testing for food allergies and sensitivities isn't one of them. While celiac disease can be quite serious, is relatively common, and has been studied extensively, there is still limited awareness of the issue among medical doctors, and the testing remains sketchy and/or inaccurate.

Given the confusion around symptoms and testing for wheat and dairy reactions, consider corn and soy, which are added in small or large quantities to most prepared foods, supplements, preservatives, and personal care products. Corn and soy are much more difficult to eliminate from the diet and personal care products, and they particularly affect glands and hormones of the complicated, non-centralized endocrine system. Gluten and dairy reactions have been studied extensively, but soy and especially corn have received minimal attention. Accurate laboratory testing for corn and soy reactions is even less likely than for gluten.

Recognizing the scope of the limitations of laboratory testing for food reactions, gut health, hormones, nutritional deficiencies, etcetera, we see the potential power of instant accurate feedback through a patient's nervous system. I don't know of other forms of manual muscle testing or other techniques that accurately and efficiently answer these questions. It is a challenging situation to recognize that my system is a significant breakthrough in healthcare, which is known fully only to me, those in my practice, and to my patients who have watched many other patients follow the Protocol and who also recognize it is unprecedented to achieve consistent results with a full spectrum of conditions. If I don't tell you this is a breakthrough, who will? My testing is deceptively simple—using touch, taste, and muscle strength—but reveals massive blind spots in healthcare. Considering the natural perfection of the body, the nervous system, and all of our senses, why wouldn't we ourselves contain the greatest potential for clear and useful answers about our own health?

The inability of laboratory tests to accurately identify reactions to gluten has led to confusion and bickering. While more medical doctors advise their patients to eliminate it from the diet, many still dismiss gluten-free diets as a fad. This rarely lands well with those of us who have confirmed that eliminating gluten eliminates many symptoms for many people.

It's often suggested that only a small percentage of the population reacts to gluten, but I find that even among young people, it is quite common, and as we age the sensitivity becomes more likely. Those currently without gluten-related symptoms may not be motivated to avoid it. But if one has significant symptoms and previously tried a gluten-free diet without improvement, it's likely worthwhile to clear intestinal infection while addressing a few other issues to confirm the negative reaction.

Avoiding gluten can be easy or difficult depending on how it's viewed. Gluten is in wheat, spelt, barley, and rye, so mostly it's about avoiding normal bread, pasta, cookies, cakes, cereal, and pizza. Tragic as this may be at times (I do miss traditional pizza), if one feels better and finds good alternatives, it doesn't mean life is over. These foods are high in carbohydrates to begin with, so making gluten-free versions often means using some other grain such as rice that may be gluten-free but is still primarily carbs. It is helpful that so many gluten-free products now exist, but most of them contain a lot of starch, which can only be absorbed as sugar and/or they contain corn in the form of xanthan gum or baking powder.

People with extreme gluten sensitivity cannot consume even trace amounts and may report that drinking distilled spirits made from glutenous grains causes negative symptoms. Most people with normal gluten sensitivity mainly avoid the obvious sources of gluten, and in time they're able to determine how much they can tolerate.

I give the following to new patients to help them identify and avoid gluten:

Gluten Avoidance

Avoid grains containing gluten: wheat, barley, rye, spelt, and anything made from these grains including bleached flour, unbleached flour, all-purpose flour, whole wheat flour, unspecified flour, sprouted wheat, wheat berries, wheat bran, wheat germ, wheatgrass, wheat gluten, bulgur, couscous, tabouli, farina, hydrolyzed wheat protein, modified food starch, semolina, durum, triticale, and Kamut. Oats in the U.S. are usually contaminated with gluten during storage and transport. There are gluten-free oats and Irish oats that are probably okay.

The following foods normally contain gluten (some come

in gluten-free versions, which may or may not be healthy food): pasta, noodles, bread, croutons, stuffing, cake, pastries, cookies, crackers, communion wafers, pretzels, crepes, breakfast cereal, pizza, falafel, candy, licorice, play dough, gravy, marinade, lunch meat, hotdogs, jerky, soy sauce, beer, anything breaded and fried (fish, chicken, calamari, etc.), malt, caramel color, MSG (monosodium glutamate), modified food starch, hydrolyzed vegetable protein, supplements, drugs, and more.

Gluten-free products are usually made from other high-carbohydrate foods, such as rice, garbanzo beans, potatoes, quinoa, buckwheat, sorghum, tapioca, etcetera. While these may be okay for an occasional treat, frequent consumption is an obstacle to optimal health. More problematic is that many gluten-free products contain ingredients usually made from corn (xanthan gum, citric acid, ascorbic acid, white vinegar, alcohol, baking powder, corn oil, etc.) or soy (soy lecithin, soy sauce, vitamin E, tocopherols, soy oil, etc.) or cow dairy products (powdered milk, whey, cream, etc.). If you know you don't react to corn, soy, or cow dairy, you might choose to eat those foods, but most people either react to them and are unaware of the reaction or will probably start to react to those foods at some point. It's best to avoid these ingredients. More companies now make better products with just a few simple ingredients and/or less sugar.

Soy

While negative reaction to soy is perhaps as common as dairy and gluten, it's minimally recognized, perhaps because soy is added to more foods, supplements, and personal care products, making it more difficult to avoid, and therefore, people are less likely to eliminate it. Even small amounts of soy can trigger significant symptoms. Some forms of soy are fairly obvious, such as soy milk, tempeh, or many items in some Asian restaurants: soy sauce, tofu, edamame, miso, teriyaki, and other sauces. However, most exposure comes from things cooked in soy oil (often called "vegetable oil"), or mayonnaise, which is usually primarily soy oil, or from food additives like lecithin, synthetic vitamin E, or tocopherols. Lecithin is added to products to make them smooth. This includes most, but not all, chocolate bars, many baked goods, and packaged foods. Vitamin E or the various forms of tocopherols somehow manage to be both a preservative and a supposed vitamin. Soy is usually found in skin lotion, sunscreen, shampoo, disposable diapers, dryer sheets, dog food, lip balm, fortified foods, most supplements, virtually all multivitamins, and some facial tissue. While there are good alternatives to these products, it takes effort to avoid soy.

Like all food reactions, soy causes symptoms relating to digestion, inflammation, headaches, skin, etcetera, but it specifically impacts the thyroid and may interfere with its ability to use iodine. The epidemic of thyroid conditions is at least partially driven by this food irritant. I find most patients benefit from a food-source iodine supplement, such as those made from kelp or other seaweed. Unfortunately, most iodine supplements are not from a food source, and alternative health practitioners tend to recommend an unnecessarily high dosage. If soy is eliminated from the diet, and a moderate amount of food-based iodine is supplemented, and the basic pieces of the Protocol are in place, then average thyroid issues disappear. However, people have to be careful when trying to discontinue a pharmaceutical, and they probably will not be able to do so if they have lost all thyroid function. This cannot be taken lightly as some people, even under ideal conditions, will have a crash of energy or mood if they stop pharmaceuticals for the thyroid. Getting off of a pharmaceutical should be done with the help of a willing medical doctor. I discuss thyroid issues further in Chapter 12.

When soy stresses the thyroid, the teres minor muscle (Figure 5 below) of the rotator cuff is weakened. This can cause shoulder issues, pain, and instability. Additionally, most carpal-tunnel-like

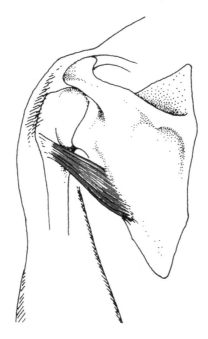

5. Teres Minor. On the back of the shoulder.

symptoms or persistent cold, numb, tingling hands and/or feet are caused or exacerbated by soy exposure. Other issues include difficulties with temperature regulation, hot flashes in women and men, mouth sores, and acne. I discuss some of these issues further in Chapters 12 and 14.

I give the following to new patients to help them identify and avoid soy:

SOY AVOIDANCE

Avoid foods made from soybeans: tofu, miso, edamame, tempeh, seitan, soy sauce, soy aminos, soy oil, vegetable oil, soy protein, soy nuts, soy milk, soy sprouts, soy lecithin (which may just be called lecithin), tocopherols or alpha tocopherols (vitamin E), MSG (monosodium glutamate), glycerin, hydrolyzed vegetable protein (HVP), and textured vegetable protein (TVP).

Foods that usually or possibly contain soy: mayonnaise, margarine, movie theater "butter," ice cream, salad dressing, cheap olive oil, artificial cheese (often used on cheap pizza), teriyaki, sushi roll sauces, jerky, BBQ sauce, carob products, meat substitutes, most chocolate bars and chocolate chips, protein/energy/candy bars or drinks, and most corporate, restaurant, prepared, and deep-fried foods.

Non-food sources of soy: skin lotion, face cream, sunscreen, chapstick, shampoo, conditioner, fabric softener, diapers, laundry detergent, and some facial tissue.

Soy-free products: soy-free chocolate bars and chocolate chips (Equal Exchange is probably the most widely available), cocoa powder, coconut aminos (soy sauce substitute), mayonnaise made from canola, safflower, or avocado oil, and miso made from garbanzo beans or other non-soy beans. Lemonaise mayonnaise contains vinegar that appears to be corn-free.

Corn

Well, if the previous three foods weren't enough bad news—or good news depending on how you look at it—corn should do the trick. Corn is everywhere. Certainly, there are corn tortillas, corn chips, popcorn, corn on the cob, and good old corn syrup, but it's with the additives where things get crazy. Corn is the number one subsidized food in the U.S., so many things like sugar, oil, vitamins, preservatives, coloring, thickeners, alcohol, and vinegar are cheapest when made from corn. Ascorbic acid, which is almost always made from corn, is a synthetic version of vitamin C that goes into sports drinks, packaged electrolytes, fortified foods, most supplements, virtually all multivitamins, and is frequently used as a preservative. While citric acid was initially identified in citrus, it's cheaper to make it from corn. Citric acid is in most canned tomatoes and sauce, canned vegetables and canned fruit, most tasty beverages in the cooler, most "natural" personal care products that aren't petroleum-based, and so on. Xanthan gum, in most gluten-free baked goods, many sauces, and other products, is usually made from corn.

Alcohol, grain alcohol, or drinking alcohol is usually made from corn and is often in herbal tinctures, beer, wine, or other alcoholic beverages, which for some reason don't have to disclose their ingredients. Bourbon has to be made from at least 51 percent corn. Most white vinegar in the U.S. is made from corn, which goes into most ketchup, mustard, pickles, hot sauce, and many other products. Alcohol is used as a solvent in the process of making a variety of pharmaceuticals, extracts such as vanilla, CBD oil, and some essential oils. Sometimes these items test well within my system, but usually the residue of corn or solvents can be identified and is problematic.

Unfortunately, corn isn't medically considered to be one of the main common allergens in the U.S., and people with this allergy or sensitivity struggle to avoid corn completely. This is partly because it's in most products and also because allergists and others suggest that as a true allergy a person reacts only to the proteins in corn. People are told that highly processed corn, which contains no proteins, is no longer corn. However, it becomes apparent that people who are sensitive to corn usually react to additives or preservatives such as citric acid, ascorbic acid (so-called "vitamin C"), white vinegar, and alcohol that are made from corn yet contain little or no corn proteins. Extremely corn-sensitive people react to things as unlikely as particular brands of bottled water, corn-based disinfectants, meat or eggs from animals who were fed corn, and the wax on commercial produce. Fortunately, this level of sensitivity is quite rare and can usually be reduced.

My testing and the symptoms that resolve when corn is eliminated from the diet make it apparent that corn sensitivity particularly affects the brain and the pituitary gland. Because the pituitary helps regulate all the glands of the body, dysfunction can contribute to any glandular or hormonal issue. The impact of corn on mental health conditions can be profound. I worked with a family who had previously tried a few times to get off of their bipolar meds. Once they eliminated corn from the diet, they no longer needed the meds. I've worked with kids and adults with ADD/ADHD whose conditions completely turned around when they eliminated corn. There were additional factors, and one should always consult a medical doctor before reducing or discontinuing a medication. Most of the time it's milder symptoms of foggy head or mild depression that come and go with exposure to corn, but many "brain chemistry" issues and dementia may be connected to the effects of corn.

The supraspinatus muscle of the rotator cuff, located on top of the shoulder (Figure 6 next page), has an association with the pituitary gland, which can be demonstrated with my technique. The pituitary, the first cervical vertebra at the top of the neck, and the TMJ (temporomandibular joint of the jaw) are closely associated. Therefore, most chronic TMJ and many shoulder joint and upper cervical issues have a strong association with reaction to corn. This pattern also creates weakness of the wrist flexors, causing tension in the opposing extensors, which frequently causes elbow and wrist conditions, including tennis elbow.

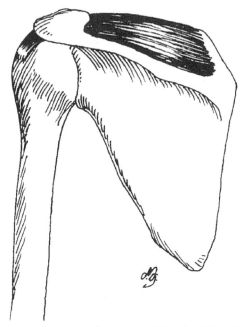

6. *Supraspinatus. On the top and back of the shoulder.*

Many chiropractors are aware of the Lovett Brother Relationship that suggests that when there is an issue with the vertebra at the top of the neck (C1) there will be a corresponding issue at the base of the spine (L5). When a patient who is sensitive to corn has consumed it in the few days before an office visit, a previously strong muscle will weaken when they touch the skin over C1 or L5, suggesting an adjustment or some form of therapy may be needed. Addressing issues with these two vertebrae is the main focus of many chiropractors, and these segments are associated with more physical symptoms than any other parts of the spine.

While many chiropractors will adjust these segments at every office visit, I find that avoiding corn is one of the most significant factors for resolving issues with these areas.

Recently, I worked with a patient who was suffering from a significant low back injury with an MRI-confirmed disc herniation. As a small business owner, he was unable to take time off from the physically demanding work that had caused the injury in the first place. After our first two visits, he was about 75 percent improved and had started to confirm that his low back pain and nerve compression pain that went to the bottom of his foot were worse with corn exposure. He continued to improve for a couple of months even though he was unable to make the two-hour trip to see me at the office. Then, his condition regressed for about three weeks until he realized that that was precisely when his sea salt had run out and he had gone back to normal table salt that contains dextrose made from corn. Four or five days later, his condition was back to dramatically improved. He still had a herniated disc, but carefully avoiding corn while following the Protocol made it possible for him to continue to heal while continuing to work.

Corn is the most difficult food irritant to avoid and has the widest range of specific symptoms associated with its consumption. While dairy and gluten and, to a lesser degree, soy are commonly recognized as allergens or irritants, corn is likely to be a larger problem. Considering the impact on personality, mood, intellect, and hormonal controls, plus the other more structural issues, the implications in a huge variety of conditions are alarming. Careful study of corn and its impacts won't be an easy task.

Two other conditions contribute to pituitary weakness: zinc deficiency and liver congestion caused by intestinal infection, issues which almost everyone has. Without addressing these two additional components while eliminating corn, it would be more difficult to achieve clear results. By addressing these, an individual's sensitivity to corn decreases. There have been some studies on ADD and a "few-food diet" that have shown encouraging results. I think this is largely due to the elimination of corn, but the reduction of carbohydrates, soy, dairy, and gluten has to help as well. At least one of these studies included wheat in the few foods that the study subjects could eat, and since wheat flour is often fortified with synthetic vitamins, which include corn-based chemicals (synthetic vitamins A and C and others), a better result could be achieved by eating meat, eggs, vegetables, and a small amounts of fruit and nuts. Corn reaction is described further in the pituitary section of Chapter 12.

I give the following to new patients to help them identify and avoid corn:

Corn Avoidance

Avoid corn-based foods: whole corn, corn on the cob, corn chips, popcorn, corn tortillas, cornbread, cornmeal, polenta, tamales, corn masa, corn starch, corn syrup, high-fructose corn syrup, corn oil, corn cereals, corn-breaded food, corn sugar, hominy (pozole), grits, corn flour, sorbitol, and corn alcohol, which is sometimes added to herbal tinctures, beer, wine, liquor, etc..

Watch out for products that usually or possibly contain corn (check ingredients): candy, baking powder, vanilla extract, herbal extracts, CBD oil, ethanol, alcohol, grain alcohol, jam, canned tomato products and other vegetables, vinegar, white vinegar, distilled white vinegar, ketchup, mustard, pickles, soda water, tonic water, most sweet drinks in a jar, fruit juice in a jar, vegetable juice in a jar, bourbon (always at least

51 percent corn), vodka (not always corn), gin (always tests poorly), soy milk, most vitamins and supplements, vitamin C, ascorbic acid, ascorbate, citric acid, citrate (often combined with minerals in supplements), vitamin E, tocopherols, vitamin A, retinyl palmitate, caramel color, artificial sweetener, xylitol, breath mints, baker's yeast, fructose, glucose, dextrose (often in table salt), maltodextrin, xanthan gum (in gluten-free products), glycerin, powdered sugar, and sugar (as an ingredient can be corn sugar, beet sugar, or cane sugar), and most corporate, restaurant, packaged, deep-fried food.

Non-foods that may contain corn: chewing gum, pharmaceuticals (over the counter and prescription), paper cups coated with cornstarch, adhesive on envelopes and stamps, body powder, clothes starch, soap, shampoo, conditioner, toothpaste, and deodorant.

Corn-free products - while they do exist, they can be hard to find: xylitol (can be made from birch or other tree bark, but rare), stevia (NOW brand), xanthan gum (Bob's Red Mill—corn-free?), baking powder (Hain), mustard and BBQ sauce made with apple cider vinegar, pickles made without white vinegar, spaghetti sauce (Kirkland organic and others), and some distilled spirits (tequila, Scotch and Irish Whiskey, and some special vodkas).

Personal Care and Household Products

Once people realize they react negatively to corn and soy, and if they also think it's a bad idea to use personal care products, household products, or supplements made from synthetic chemicals and petroleum products, then we start to realize there are very few of these products we want to bring into our homes. If there are too many problematic, complicated chemical names listed or if one is reluctant to eat or at least taste a product, it probably shouldn't go on the skin or in the body. There is almost nothing at a major drug store that fits these guidelines. Even at a good health food store most "natural" products are preserved with citric acid or tocopherols that are made from corn or soy or they contain corn alcohol, glycerin, xanthan gum, or other problematic chemicals. While some companies can be helpful in the disclosure of the sources of their product ingredients, many either don't know or won't reply to inquiries, and ingredients often change, especially with smaller companies.

With these problems it is incredibly valuable to be able to test products directly through sense of taste and accurate muscle testing. For example, I didn't realize that CBD oil made from cannabis usually contains residual corn alcohol until I had tested a few people to the products they were using and then did a little research. I never would have thought that the balsamic vinegar from the big chain gourmet store contained either corn or chemicals until it became obvious through testing, elimination, and subsequent resolution of symptoms. While it may be awkward at a party, it is amazing to observe that most California wines test poorly because of undisclosed additives, but most European wines test well. It is astounding to see the frequency with which patients suffer symptoms from trying various supplements that usually contain corn, soy, or chemicals.

While learning how to carefully read ingredient lists is essential, it doesn't always give the full story, and early in care patients often slip up. If a patient isn't achieving great results with the Protocol and all of the main indicators test well, I will suggest they bring in any products they are using that are questionable. Often, we discover the obstacle to their success.

I would like to be able to give a list of ingredients that are okay and those to avoid, but there are too many possibilities and too many exceptions. For example, citrate usually is citric acid from GMO corn that is combined with other things such as magnesium to form supplements like magnesium citrate. Most magnesium citrate supplements test poorly for people who are sensitive to corn. However, the calcium lactate supplement that I use contains magnesium citrate and it tests well, and the product works well even with people who are very sensitive to corn. I don't know if that citrate comes from corn. If it does, it is processed in a way that removes the offending factor, whatever that is. Sometimes companies will tell us that something is made from corn or soy, but it is processed such that there are no proteins remaining or that it is no longer considered corn or soy. For particular products, my testing agrees with that statement, and with others, it doesn't. I use a lysine supplement that claims to contain soy, but people never test poorly to it, and I have never seen a soy-sensitive patient, or any patient, react negatively to it.

Another problem is that people can develop secondary sensitivities to almost anything when chronic intestinal infection and leaky gut are present. There are those who experience symptoms or have health concerns about ingredients such as canola oil, guar gum, carrageenan, calcium stearate, magnesium stearate, palm oil, and others. While I may prefer simpler ingredients or alternatives to these, and while some forms of these ingredients may test poorly depending on their source and processing, in certain forms in certain products I consume these with confidence. However, any products that we bring home with these ingredients we test if we will be eating it or using it much. We also avoid products with known ecological or social justice issues.

I have a list at theprotocolforhealth.com of products or supplements that I use, recommend, and/or sell that test and work well within my system. I plan to keep adding to that list. Unfortunately, things will likely be removed from that list as products change, companies are sold, and manufacturers choose cheaper ingredients.

TREE NUT SENSITIVITY

While not as common as the previous four reactions, sensitivity to tree nuts and almonds in particular seems to be increasing. Nuts may or may not cause typical symptoms of sensitivity such as issues with digestion, skin, headaches, sinus congestion, etcetera. I often discover this sensitivity by first identifying weakness of the small neck flexor muscles—the anterior scalenes. I then test the patient to nuts through sense of taste, usually confirming this sensitivity. Problematic chemical exposure or other sensitivities can also cause weak scalenes, but reaction to nuts is most common. A few days after removing nuts from the diet, the weakness resolves. When this muscle weakness is present, it often causes pain or other symptoms of the head, neck, shoulders, arms, and/or hands that resolve with the dietary change. Sensitivity to nuts is rare enough that I don't suggest that most of my patients remove them from the diet unless we confirm the reaction. With patients who are particularly compromised, it's often safer to avoid nuts until they are less reactive in general. Most—but certainly not everyone—can eventually bring nuts back into the diet. If they are consumed excessively, in less pure forms, or in conjunction with chronic intestinal infection, the reaction may develop. Organic versus nonorganic seems to be particularly important with nuts in general and almonds in particular.

CHAPTER 6
The Third Cause of Disease and the Unexpected Solution

Adrenal Fatigue, Blood Sugar Instability, and Elevated Cortisol

Years ago, when my wife and I had moved out of the honeymoon phase of our relationship, we found ourselves sometimes arguing about nothing at the end of the day. I started calling timeout to ask what we had eaten for breakfast that morning. It became obvious that pointless arguments at the end of the day usually followed a morning where coffee on an empty stomach or birthday cake for breakfast seemed like a good idea. Now we eat a protein breakfast with little or no sugar or starch, and if there's caffeine, it only comes right after breakfast. Not only have we avoided most of the arguments about nothing, but we sleep better, have better energy in general, and the knee problems that plagued me for years are gone. It's not always easy for our daughters to be positive about a weekend breakfast without maple syrup, so we compromise sometimes, but in general, low-carb, protein-based breakfasts contribute to their mental, emotional, and physical stability.

Blood sugar instability or relying on the adrenal glands to regulate blood sugar is one of the seven main causes of pain and disease. It's a result of normal lifestyles in the U.S. and most industrialized nations. It's caused by eating sugar or starch on an empty stomach or from being active or drinking caffeine without first having a protein-based meal to stabilize and fuel the body. Under these conditions the adrenal glands release cortisol to raise blood sugar and fuel activity. While the body can do this for some time, perhaps decades in otherwise healthy individuals, eventually symptoms result. There's a cost for relying on small glands to stabilize blood sugar rather than maintaining stability through the diet.

It's important to remember that we're talking about the available energy for every cell in the body and for every function performed. It's much easier to create health and a stable life when the blood sugar is stable. Before looking to techniques that offer "cellular healing" or "reprogramming" or the latest pharmaceutical, it's helpful to make sure our cells have a sustainable energy source, also known as breakfast, lunch, and dinner and a couple of snacks.

For breakfast, I usually have eggs and quality ham. I eat vegetables later in the day so I can get right to a reasonable cup of 50/50 regular/decaf organic coffee. There are many other versions of a decent breakfast, and including vegetables at breakfast can be helpful, for some.

If blood sugar isn't kept stable with frequent protein-based meals, then it's up to the adrenals to make an abundance of cortisol to keep us going. Eventually this will stress the adrenals and cause muscle weakness. Issues related directly to adrenal fatigue include inability to stay asleep for eight hours, fatigue and/or crankiness, especially in the afternoon or early evening, chronic knee pain, ligament laxity, and structural tissue failures such as hernias, hemorrhoids (also caused by liver congestion), and torn tendons. Additionally, headaches, low back pain, and some hormonal problems may be caused by blood sugar instability, but these complaints often have other, more significant factors. Chronically elevated cortisol is known to increase inflammation, interfere with healing of wounds and tissues (skin, gut lining, liver, cartilage, brain, etc.), compromise immune function, decrease bone formation, decrease appetite, and contribute to weight gain and premature aging. Skipping breakfast for a cup of coffee could eventually become extremely uncomfortable and/or expensive.

Blood sugar instability often results from not eating because of weak stomach acid and low appetite, not making time for meals, fasting while being active, eating meals consisting primarily of carbohydrates, eating inadequate protein, over-consuming stimulants, and consuming stimulants on an empty stomach.

Generally, people think of the adrenal glands making adrenalin for fight-or-flight reactions, but the main product of the adrenals is cortisol, which has the primary purpose of elevating blood sugar. Cortisol is also elevated in response to physical and emotional stress. Using these glands to respond to stress and to compensate for frequent swings in blood sugar eventually stresses the adrenals and causes symptoms.

While adrenal fatigue and symptoms of high cortisol are big topics in mainstream and alternative medicine, the solution is much simpler than most realize. If the blood sugar is kept stable through diet and mindful timing of the diet, the vast majority of adrenal and cortisol issues disappear. By addressing the main physical stresses (the six other causes of disease) and keeping blood sugar stable, it becomes apparent that emotional stress is not the real driver of adrenal fatigue or other symptoms, pain, and disease.

Emotional stress exacerbates underlying issues. When we address the underlying issues, emotional stress becomes easier to manage and physical symptoms decrease. A history of trauma and prolonged serious emotional stress is associated with an increased risk of a wide variety of conditions. Chronic stress that chronically compromises our ability to make stomach acid combined with blood sugar instability that elevates cortisol is likely the main reason for this link between stress and disease. Many people can't really eat or eat well when they're stressed, so the blood sugar becomes unstable and cortisol is elevated. If this goes on for too long, weak stomach acid leads to poor absorption, vitamin and mineral deficiencies, and chronic intestinal infection and the associated issues.

I give the following directions to new patients to help them stabilize blood sugar:

> BLOOD SUGAR STABILITY—ADRENAL SUPPORT GUIDELINES
>
> The goal is to maintain stable blood sugar and avoid spikes and crashes. When stability is achieved, the adrenal glands no longer need to compensate for these swings, and adrenal function usually normalizes.
>
> - Ingest caffeine in moderation only* and only right after eating protein.
> - Don't ingest caffeine before breakfast or more than one hour after eating protein.
> - Limit physical activity before breakfast to less than the equivalent of taking a shower.
> - Eat a minimum of fifteen grams** of protein within thirty minutes of rising in the morning.
> - Don't go more than three hours after a full meal without eating a protein snack during the busy part of the day.
> - Eating a protein snack (seven-gram minimum) buys you one-and-a-half to two hours before your next meal.
> - Eat a minimum of fifteen grams* of protein at lunch.
> - Continue frequent protein during the busy, active, stressful part of the day.

- Limit caffeine to one reasonable cup per day. If there is a second dose of caffeine, it should be small and only occasional.
- Know that as we age, we become more sensitive to caffeine.
- Consider 50/50 regular/decaf organic coffee. Decaf contains up to one-third of the caffeine.
- Avoid decaf, chocolate, and caffeine four-plus hours before bed to ensure better sleep.

Good sources of protein are meat, poultry, fish, and eggs. If your digestion and elimination are very good (no diarrhea or discomfort), you might include nuts or nut butters. Significant quantities of nuts may cause weight gain or digestive disturbance, and those with especially compromised health may need to avoid nuts. Goat or water buffalo milk products are good protein sources for most people but may cause weight gain. Most react negatively to cow's milk dairy products but don't recognize its symptoms. Avoid it for at least the first two months of the Protocol.

* If your condition is more advanced (diabetes, etc.), or you want to eat more carefully, you might eliminate caffeine and alcohol as well as most carbohydrates. However, it's better to include these things in moderation and succeed on the other more important aspects of the Protocol than to deprive yourself of caffeine and/or alcohol and be overwhelmed and give up.

** Fifteen grams of protein is equivalent to two extra-large eggs or a little more than two ounces of meat or goat cheese or four tablespoons of nut butter. Fifteen grams is a minimum. An individual's age, size, and activity might indicate two to four times that amount.

If you don't eat protein in the morning before activity, or you go too long without protein during the day, or consume sugar or caffeine on an empty stomach, the adrenal glands compensate for what is being asked of the body. While the adrenals can manage this for some time without adverse effects, at some point unstable blood sugar, which causes elevated cortisol, becomes overly stressful and symptoms result.

After going all night without food, our blood sugar is likely at its lowest daily level, and cortisol is usually at its highest. If we start our morning with caffeine, this stimulant demands activity of the body, but without food, we lack the immediate fuel to deliver on that demand, so the adrenals release more cortisol. Also, if we don't have breakfast soon after rising, the adrenals must supply cortisol for even mild activities, such as taking a shower, let alone exercising, or going for a run. If we do eat breakfast, but it consists only of carbohydrates (sugar and starch), such as fruit, bread, cereal, oatmeal, or maybe a donut, then the blood sugar spikes and crashes soon after, and the adrenals compensate for the inadequate breakfast. Or maybe we eat a solid breakfast, like eggs and meat, but if it's finished at seven o'clock and lunch is at noon or later, that food or fuel runs out after about three hours, and the adrenals keep us going until we eat again. The same is true with lunch at noon and not eating again until seven or eight in the evening, and maybe we have a beer before dinner, which spikes the blood sugar. All of these scenarios result in small glands keeping us active rather than feeding ourselves in a manner that keeps the blood sugar stable.

The adrenals have an association with three muscles that cross the knee. Two of these muscles also cross the hip, the gracilis and sartorius, and the other crosses the ankle, the gastrocnemius or calf muscle (Figures 7, 8, and 9 respectively, pages 109 and 110). When the adrenals are stressed, these muscles weaken and cause opposing muscle tension. This imbalance compromises the movement and tracking of the knees and hips and makes them vulnerable to injury, harder to heal, and may cause the body to grind away its own cartilage, which then fails to heal because of elevated cortisol, inflammation, and poor absorption. Muscle imbalance may cause pain on its own, but the imbalance also makes us vulnerable such that even a minor accident may tear muscles, tendons, ligaments, or cartilage. The combination of elevated cortisol, muscle imbalance, inflammation, and poor absorption of nutrients sets conditions for pain, inflammation, arthritis, and degeneration that has resulted in about five million Americans currently living with knee replacements, and 2.5 million with hip replacements.

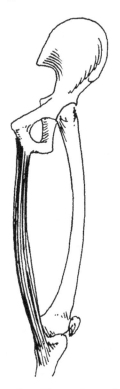 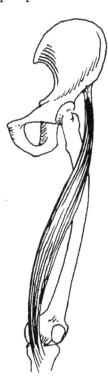

7. *Gracilis. From the pelvis to below the knee (rotated out).*

8. *Sartorius. From the pelvis to below the knee (rotated out).*

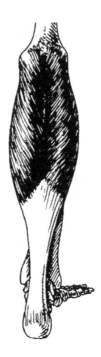

9. Gastrocnemius. From the back of the knee to the heel.

Frequently, new patients complain of the combination of inability to sleep for eight hours, low energy, and moodiness combined with chronic hip or knee pain. By following the Protocol and particularly the adrenal diet, these issues generally resolve within two to eight weeks. Knees usually heal faster than hips, and hips usually have more complicating factors. In this process energy increases as sleep improves and patients get off the roller coaster of blood sugar and cortisol swings. While it may seem strange that knee problems could be caused simply by blood sugar instability, using this protocol leaves me and my patients with little doubt. If someone complains of chronic knee pain or instability (and serious, immediate issues have been ruled out), pain improves or goes away by following the Blood Sugar Stability—Adrenal Support Guidelines.

A patient I hadn't seen for a few months called me with bad

knee pain. She lives a few hours away and was unable to come see me at the time. She was about to go see an orthopedic surgeon about her pain. I asked how she was eating, and it turned out she was doing some sort of fasting cleanse. I reminded her of the diet. She called me two days later to report her pain was gone. A study to show the consistency of this solution would be great, and I'd bet more than half of knee replacements could be avoided this way.

The other group of patients who respond well to stabilizing the blood sugar are those who, upon describing their condition at our first visit, break into tears. Emotional overwhelm and sensitivity often ease profoundly by following these guidelines. Blood sugar instability may present itself as sensitivity, irritability, depression, or exhaustion. Many factors contribute to these issues, but with tears on a first visit, blood sugar stability is usually a life changer. Most people taking mood-altering drugs improve significantly with this solution.

Many alternative health authors and practitioners claim that one needs to eliminate stress from life, play soothing music, get more hugs, meditate two hours a day, and maybe live in a cave— all of which may be nice or helpful, and some of which aren't really possible.

We were built for stress, and while stress exacerbates many conditions, clearing underlying physical stress usually eliminates physical symptoms from all types of stress. Or you could say the biggest stress most people suffer from is the physical stress of relying on the adrenals to maintain blood sugar stability and the associated elevated cortisol.

While chronically elevated cortisol is known to drive many symptoms, most studies on reducing cortisol look at treatments such as music, laughter, dance, herbs, or other peripheral solutions. Cortisol is a glucocorticoid, a steroid hormone with the primary purpose of elevating blood glucose or maintaining blood sugar levels. It's the primary product of the adrenals. If a patient has stressed adrenals and elevated cortisol, it's sensible to stabilize blood sugar with a careful diet of frequent protein that takes pressure off the adrenals and decreases cortisol levels.

While I'm describing this aspect of the Protocol in terms of blood sugar and cortisol levels, this is a working model to describe the process. I never actually order laboratory work for blood sugar or cortisol. This model describes the internal conditions addressed by a dietary solution. It's identified through patterns of muscle weakness and cross-checked to reflex points, which all resolve along with symptoms when the Adrenal Support diet is followed. Ordering blood work to confirm this model would be expensive, impractical, and/or inaccurate because the normal fluctuation of cortisol over twenty-four hours would require multiple tests per day before and after the dietary changes.

My testing identifies whether or not the adrenals are stressed by the recent diet and lifestyle habits of an individual. When people follow the Adrenal Support diet, the indicators and symptoms clear quickly. The Protocol works so consistently that if someone didn't improve as expected, I would refer them to the appropriate disease specialist to be co-managed as needed. So far, I haven't had to do that.

Appetite, Eating, and Absorption

Unfortunately, some common obstacles make it difficult for many to eat protein frequently. Most people have weak stomach acid, intestinal infection, adrenal fatigue, and elevated cortisol. All of these factors interfere with digestion and may suppress the appetite. Drinking too much coffee, going without breakfast or too long without eating elevates cortisol, which engages fight-or-flight or the sympathetic nervous system and suppresses rest-

and-digest, the parasympathetic nervous system and therefore, a healthy appetite. Making time for adequate, mild aerobic exercise, while not overdoing it on anaerobic exercise (Chapter 9) and keeping carbohydrates relatively low (Chapter 8) are also essential to lowering cortisol. If people with blood sugar stability issues "listen to their body" and only eat when they're hungry, the issue persists. The appetite is low because of weak stomach acid and elevated cortisol.

Sometimes this unhealthy cycle is broken simply by following the Blood Sugar Stability Guidelines—eating protein frequently, even if not hungry—and often the appetite improves, and people start to wake ready for food. Some can't improve appetite until digestion is addressed, and without that, they may find it uncomfortable or impossible to eat frequently. This sets up conditions for losing muscle mass and aging prematurely. However, when eating frequently, gaining body fat can be a problem if too much of the wrong foods are consumed.

For people who can't eat adequately and/or gain weight, such as children who aren't growing effectively, elderly patients who are losing muscle mass, pregnant women with nausea, or patients with no appetite because of cancer treatments, this approach can change their medical future. Creating a healthy appetite and improving absorption of nutrients can enable people of any age to gain muscle mass and dramatically improve their health.

One great example of this is a patient in his seventies who found he could hand dig a large French drain in his backyard all summer after we cleared his intestinal pain, kidney issues, and recurring infections. These were considered to be complications of Agent Orange exposure from fifty years prior. By the end of the summer, he had gained significant muscle mass, which was previously impossible. I've also worked with guys in their twenties who put on more than twenty pounds of muscle in the few months after they started the Protocol. I worked with a teenager who was receiving cancer treatments and was the only kid in the children's cancer ward sitting up and asking for more food. These results are possible not because of a simple pill or therapy, but because of the seven components of the Protocol for Health.

An extremely poor appetite is called anorexia. While that's not the same as the eating disorder anorexia nervosa, strengthening digestion, improving absorption, and decreasing any negative physical symptoms associated with eating and digestion are helpful for both conditions. Those who are sensitive to the smells of certain foods, only eat certain things or only a few bites, or who just don't like eating are usually more able to eat a full and varied diet with this approach. I don't treat mental health issues but removing physical obstacles and reducing physical stress allows people more space for working on a variety of issues. Sleeping better, having more energy, and feeling better overall improves our chances of addressing any issue.

INTERMITTENT FASTING? THERE IS A BETTER SOLUTION.

Intermittent fasting has recently become the most popular dietary technique. While there are many different forms, it comes down to not eating for certain periods of time. I explore this topic in detail because fasting while being active is opposite to the Adrenal Support diet I recommend, and while intermittent fasting sometimes helps to control symptoms or to achieve certain goals, I see it cause stress, weakness, and eventual breakdown, and it fails to address causative issues. When the Protocol for Health is applied, underlying issues are addressed so that better health can be achieved without intermittent fasting. Because of common issues, intermittent fasting helps many feel better, but it doesn't create conditions for optimal sustained health.

One such common issue is weak stomach acid. People with inadequate stomach acid due to zinc deficiency and elevated cortisol may feel better if they take a break from eating or engage in intermittent fasting. In this way they save limited, precious stomach acid for less frequent meals, but the cost is decreased nutrient consumption and therefore, decreased absorption and elevated cortisol from abstaining from protein for more than three hours while being active. This issue is resolved when zinc is adequately absorbed and utilized, and people produce adequate stomach acid to eat regularly.

A related common issue is leaky gut caused by chronic intestinal infection. For those with chronic intestinal infection, which is almost everyone, even a perfect diet allows undigested food proteins into the blood, causing inflammation after every meal. Without eating, there may be less inflammatory response (except for what's created by elevated cortisol), and the body has time to clear proteins and undigested nutrients from the blood that are there because of the underlying issue. Essentially, people with leaky gut experience repetitive stress injuries just from eating. With this condition, they may feel better for a while if they don't eat. When the underlying chronic intestinal infection is addressed, there is less inflammation after meals, so minimal recovery from a meal is required, and people can eat and feel good.

When leaky gut is addressed, the liver, gallbladder, and kidneys—the body's main systems for removing waste products—are no longer overloaded with food proteins and therefore have a greater capacity to eliminate other waste, excess hormones, heavy metals, and toxins—some of the main causes of inflammation, pain, cancer, and most health issues.

Most of us eat foods we weren't designed to eat as well as too much sugar, or too much food in general. We may feel better if we stop eating temporarily, and it also may help us lose weight. Some use intermittent fasting because they want to lose weight despite eating a less-than-optimal diet. Better and more sustainable for our health is to eat a good diet, keep the blood sugar stable, and then decide if we need to work on losing weight.

Each of these components above can make fasting look like a miracle cure in the short term; therefore, many people take this route and find it helpful because of the common underlying issues. If those issues are addressed, people can eat, feel good, and enjoy the benefits of stable blood sugar, less inflammation, and better nutrient absorption.

The goal of intermittent fasting for some is to stimulate autophagy: the body's ability to self-clean and remove cells and other components that are ready to be retired. The idea of this approach to intermittent fasting is that stress is needed to stimulate this process. Forms include not eating or not eating protein on various schedules, intentionally drinking coffee on an empty stomach, or stressing the body by performing high-intensity exercise. But if zinc absorption, stomach acid production, leaky gut/intestinal infection, and the diet are addressed, then we have completely changed the internal environment, and fasting for autophagy makes less sense.

Simply addressing zinc deficiency and elevated cortisol has the potential to significantly improve autophagy. Both zinc deficiency and elevated cortisol are known to interfere with wound and tissue healing. On a cellular level, wound healing *is* autophagy *and* healing of damaged tissue. Zinc deficiency and elevated cortisol also interfere with the absorption of nutrients needed to maintain and build the body. Autophagy may be a worthy goal, but components that are directly involved with healing and rebuilding are more important.

We don't need to add stress to the body to trick it into the normal, natural function of autophagy. Cultural anthropologists tell us that traditional hunter-gatherers spent ten to twenty hours per week attending to food and shelter under conditions where they had not been marginalized and before environmental degradation. These conditions no longer exist because of industrialization and the resulting elevated CO_2. Zinc deficiency affects all of us now and the plants and animals we eat. There was plenty of food most of the time; people, like any animal, were well adapted to their environments, and foragers didn't have to conduct fasting to be healthy. It doesn't make sense to fast to stress the body to recreate an idea about Ancestral Health that probably doesn't describe the lifestyles of most of our ancestors, most of the time, before agriculture.

High-intensity exercise may be a useful form of stress for inducing autophagy if it isn't excessive and if we have the heart and lungs to back it up. But most of us don't walk as our ancestors did, so we aren't ready for much high-intensity exercise because of our limited heart and lung capacity (Chapter 9).

The concept of stimulating autophagy through intermittent fasting seems overly complicated and unnatural. By implementing the Protocol, I think most of the claimed benefits and reasoning are addressed more holistically.

Some proponents of intermittent fasting describe that they have minimal appetite, lose weight, have tons of energy, and don't need to, or can't, sleep for eight hours. That sounds like a description of the short-term effects of elevated cortisol, weight-loss supplements, or drug stimulants. They can be sustained for some time, especially by otherwise healthy individuals, but sooner or later there will be consequences.

However, if people are done with the active part of their day by six or seven in the evening (not doing the dishes, laundry, exercise, or out on the town) and they don't eat from then until after they wake in the morning, this would be about twelve hours without eating, which would be a way to intermittent fast and follow the Protocol at the same time. I haven't seen that to be necessary, but it may be helpful for some.

There's also fasting for spiritual or other purposes. Ideally, this is accompanied by meditation or prayer and not by work, driving, and activity. It's fasting while being active that creates problems. This is contrary to some religious guidelines.

My testing can determine if fasting is stressing the adrenals and causing muscle weakness, which is what I usually find with those fasting while being active. If a person is intermittent fasting and has chronic knee pain, poor sleep, and mood swings, then the adrenals are stressed, and they will benefit from the Protocol.

While I'm confident that not eating a protein breakfast and exercising on an empty stomach will eventually cause symptoms, some can sustain that lifestyle for extended periods of time and appear to be healthy. Are their adrenals stressed? Are their knees vulnerable to injury? Are they susceptible to other issues from elevated cortisol? So far, that's what my testing has shown with extended intermittent fasting.

Once blood sugar is stable and the other pieces of the Protocol are in place, energy generally increases and, if knee pain is present, it improves. These conditions prepare people for the other important factor regarding cortisol: regular, sustained, aerobic exercise such as walking or running slowly, which I discuss in Chapter 9.

Other issues closely related to adrenal function include immunity, allergies, torn muscles, tendons, and ligaments, unexplained fractures, low bone density, weight management (gaining or losing), inflammation, bloating, endocrine issues, and hormone regulation and production, especially around menopause. These topics are explored elsewhere in this book.

CHAPTER 7
The Fourth Cause of Disease and the Unexpected Solution

Deficiencies of Basic Vitamins and Minerals

The vitamin and mineral deficiencies I find with muscle testing reflect basic nutrients known to be essential building blocks for the body: zinc, calcium, magnesium, iron/B12/B complex, iodine/trace minerals, and vitamin A. I also find a pattern of weakness and symptoms that can be addressed with a concentrated sesame oil, and often muscle injuries clear to Biost, a supplement made from red meat prepared at low temperature. These supplements combined with betaine hydrochloride (HCl) make up what I call the Basic 9, or Basic 8 if patients prefer to eat pink red meat frequently instead of Biost. These supplements essentially form a multivitamin from mostly food sources.

Of course, we would like to believe that eating a good diet and maintaining strong digestion should supply adequate nutrients from quality foods, but I don't find that. Our nutritional deficiencies are probably caused by factors more or less outside of our control such as atmospheric changes and the limitations of agriculture, as well as our modern food choices, chemical exposure, and elevated cortisol.

Testing reveals patterns of muscle weakness that correlate with reflex points and symptoms that clear when people absorb and utilize mostly food-based supplements or sometimes when they eat a lot of certain nutrient-dense foods. My patients confirm for themselves that the supplements we use to address these weaknesses are effective in terms of symptoms, strength, performance, and blood work. While some deficiencies can be addressed with specific foods, such as eating a cup of cooked beet greens daily for calcium, effective supplements with strong digestion usually work out to be less expensive and easier to take consistently.

I also use other supplements in practice: a couple for fighting acute viral infections (cold or flu-like symptoms), a couple for certain types of acute bacterial infections, rarely some for clearing liver and gallbladder congestion, and a few specific whole glandular supplements usually for short-term support of parts of the endocrine system. Compared to most alternative health practitioners, this is a short list of simple supplements, which may occur to some as overly simplistic and lacking in specificity. By addressing causes of health issues and disease, it becomes unnecessary to treat peripheral issues or peripheral deficiencies with more complicated and specialized supplements, and peripheral problems disappear as core issues are resolved. Remove the main obstacles to health and then diet, aerobic exercise, and basic supplements provide the foundation for the ultimate self-contained pharmacy.

There are many popular supplements used by alternative medicine and laypeople for digestive complaints. A variety of supplements and pharmaceuticals soothe the stomach or intestines, alter bowel movements, or control other digestive symptoms. When we strengthen stomach acid with betaine hydrochloride, use zinc to improve stomach acid production, clear chronic intestinal infection with a course of specific digestive enzymes, implement a good diet, and use a few supplements for the deficiencies most people have (what we wish a multivitamin could address), most digestive complaints clear up. This renders medications for heartburn, diarrhea, and constipation irrelevant, and many supplements unnecessary: probiotics, licorice root, L-glutamine, aloe vera, apple cider vinegar, colostrum, wormwood, black walnut, cayenne, oregano, continual digestive enzymes, diatomaceous earth, slippery elm, and psyllium husk, to name a few.

Those with pain sometimes find that chondroitin sulfate, turmeric, "vitamin" D, or omega-3 fish oil improve symptoms, but after clearing inflammation and improving nutrient absorption, patients feel better and don't miss those supplements. Some practitioners use specific supplements intended to affect neurotransmitters or the heart, eyes, brain, etcetera. Often, there is some special berry, extract, antioxidant, or mineral source people may or may not notice they benefit from taking. I consistently help people to feel better by addressing causative issues; this allows them to move away from long lists of supplements and address a few foundational deficiencies with simple supplements that can be fully utilized.

Regarding the bewildering supply of available supplements in the marketplace, the solution I've found treats causative issues first with a good diet, strong digestion, effective exercise and then addresses long-term nutritional needs with mostly food-based simple supplements. Symptoms are not caused by a lack of some powerful herb or a deficiency of an extra fancy antioxidant; those aren't causative issues. If the body can absorb nutrients effectively, which most can't, and eliminate waste products and toxins effectively, which most can't, then drinking a huge algae smoothie or taking random supplements to control symptoms becomes unnecessary. With pervasive chronic intestinal infection, it's easy to sell overly complicated, expensive cleanses and maintenance regimens that go on forever and ever. These plans may involve heavy-handed chelation therapies, invasive colonics, long-term fasting, synthetic chemicals, natural forms of poison for cleansing or clearing parasites, and powerful herbs. While these may or may not help people feel better and may possibly improve blood work and decrease significant symptoms, they don't get to the cause of health issues. Those regimens must be continued or repeated indefinitely, can't achieve a full result, likely have some negative side effects, and are more expensive over time. However, without access to a better solution, those methods may still be helpful in the short-term. Most people suffer from deficiencies and inflammation and are overloaded with waste products and chemicals they can't fully clear from the body. If one addresses even one of those issues it might be enough to delay the usual train wreck of health problems.

Actual full absorption of even the best quality supplements is not straightforward. Supplements usually aren't absorbed and utilized well enough to clear muscle weaknesses, and most people have internal issues that interfere with absorption. When people first come to see me, I suggest they at least temporarily stop taking any supplements for which they are uncertain of the benefits, as long as it's not a medical prescription. Most people report no noticeable benefit from most of their supplements, so they don't mind putting them on hold. If they know that a supplement is helping, then we keep it in place until we have addressed the underlying cause and/or moved to a simpler solution. The big studies on multivitamins show no help for our biggest issues: heart disease, cancer, and mental decline. Useful supplements combined with strong digestion and absorption actually make people feel better as well as contributing to long-term health.

I recently saw a patient who had been following the Protocol for roughly three years. I hadn't seen her for almost a year. She had had plantar fasciitis for a couple months that limited her walking. She had also been ignoring nausea after taking a handful of mostly food-based daily supplements I had recommended. With muscle testing, I confirmed she wasn't adequately absorbing the zinc she was taking and therefore was unable to make sufficient stomach acid to fully digest and absorb nutrients from her food and supplements. I helped her understand how and when to increase her betaine hydrochloride stomach acid supplement and reminded her of the protocol for lowering cortisol to improve absorption. The next morning the nausea was gone, and the plantar fasciitis resolved in another two or three days. The betaine hydrochloride enabled her to absorb the zinc to make her own stomach acid, and absorbing calcium restored her muscular endurance; strengthening the arch and taking tension off the plantar fascia. As she started to fully absorb the supplements again, her energy, mood, and overall strength also improved.

Effective absorption of simple, quality supplements is very different from most people's experiences. Supplements should not only address long-term issues but create noticeable changes within days to a couple of weeks of starting or stopping. Enabling supplement absorption illuminates solutions to many specific symptoms rarely addressed at the causative level by the full spectrum of healthcare. Osteoporosis keeps getting worse. It's caused by inadequate absorption and *utilization* of calcium and other minerals combined with hormone imbalance. Modern medicine doesn't effectively address it. Absorbing vitamin B12 under the tongue or getting B12 injections doesn't make much sense. Yes, the injections may help many symptoms, but ideally, we address why a patient can't naturally absorb B12 in the gut. When B12 is absorbed, there are many benefits for the patient and their nervous system in particular, and the associated muscle weakness that is addressed enables ankle injuries to heal and/or become less likely. Chronic fatigue is rarely treated effectively. How can one have adequate energy when barely absorbing vitamins and minerals necessary for life? Plantar fasciitis is driven by calcium deficiency. Heartburn is driven by weak stomach acid and deficiency of zinc. Leg cramps and restless leg syndrome clear when minerals are absorbed. Anxiety, panic attacks, and heartbeat irregularities get better or resolve with effective mineral absorption. Minerals in the heart allow the essential electrical impulse to travel through the muscle so the heart contracts properly. Compromised function of the heart is frightening and/or stressful and frequently drives physical and emotional anxiety. Endurance and exercise recovery time improve dramatically when even a quarter of the RDA of calcium is absorbed in a useful form. We need calcium for every muscle contraction in the body. Magnesium deficiency is linked to heart disease, perhaps more strongly than elevated cholesterol. Emergency room injections of magnesium save the lives of many heart attack victims—better to absorb it before that event. All of the solutions above are unknown, or rarely very effective, because the supplements that solve the problems are rarely fully absorbed and utilized in the tissues where they're needed.

I don't get to look inside the body and know how much a person is absorbing; my muscle tests utilizing the patient's own nervous system provide the reliable feedback I need to determine if adequate nutrients are going where they're needed, in a usable form, to clear weaknesses and related symptoms. Sometimes nutrients are absorbed but not in a form that can be utilized. This may result in blood tests that confirm a nutrient is present in the blood, but it may not contribute to improving health or reducing symptoms, or it may create negative side effects. Possibly, it's strong stomach acid that prepares a mineral for absorption or utilization in a way that weak stomach acid cannot. That most supplements are made from rocks, chemicals, and food allergens is part of the problem. Most magnesium supplements are magnesium citrate. This is magnesium chelated with citric acid usually made from GMO corn. Most people have an unrecognized sensitivity to corn or will eventually. Laboratory tests for identifying deficiencies are limited or inadequate. Considering how essential magnesium is to the beating of the heart, and that it's impossible to measure magnesium in the heart of a living person, and that only 1 percent of magnesium is in the blood, better testing for magnesium deficiency could drastically change our understanding of the role of magnesium in heart disease. Every vitamin and mineral have similar problems in the standard routes of supplementation and laboratory detection. Science and medicine are a long way from a real solution.

What supplement could be more fundamental and more carefully studied than calcium? It's the foundation of our bones, and it's needed for every muscle contraction, including the beating of our hearts. With two million fractures from osteoporosis in this country every year, and heart disease being the number one killer, these are critical issues. Modern medicine can't enable people to adequately absorb calcium, or at least not in a usable form. The story around calcium supplements has constantly changed over the years from one chelated form to another, combined with various compounds. Take it with vitamin K, take it with magnesium, and now take it with "vitamin" D. D is not a vitamin. It's a hormone that our skin makes when exposed to the sun. Adding synthetic hormones to the body carries risk, and studies don't support that supplementing with synthetic D helps people absorb calcium or build bones. Can we absorb calcium from cow's milk? Does consuming milk actually contribute to calcium deficiency? It can't even be proven that calcium supplements decrease risk of fractures. Now calcium supplements are being linked to heart disease and kidney stones. We have one of *the highest rates* of dairy consumption and calcium supplement consumption in the world, yet we have the highest rate of osteoporosis, and it's getting worse.

This isn't about criticizing modern medicine. It's important to recognize the blind spots and consider alternate means of insight. People put much faith and trust into a system that hasn't determined how to enable absorption of our most fundamental mineral. That's not to say that science and medicine should be disregarded because they can't facilitate absorption, only that this example illustrates the complexity of the body's systems and the challenge of intervening with these systems. Using the nervous system of a patient to guide treatment allows the nervous system to simplify the process. The answers come in the form of strong, weak, or no change in muscle strength. Laboratory tests can't conclusively identify which foods we should eat and which foods harm us, but under certain conditions, the nervous system can. There is no proven laboratory test for the zinc deficiency that drives all other deficiencies, but the answer is available through the nervous system. Muscle testing isn't just pushing and pulling with arms and legs; it's a route that reveals and addresses some of the biggest blind spots in healthcare. It's why I can guarantee results with so many conditions that are normally very difficult or impossible to treat.

Calcium makes up 1.4 percent of our body mass, but zinc is only .0032 percent, and iodine is .000016 percent, and yet they play critical roles in our bodies. Calcium deficiency has been studied far more than other deficiencies because it creates obvious problems in the U.S. and other industrialized nations: many bones break because of it. But despite the World Health Organization reporting a million deaths per year globally from zinc deficiency, it has less available research and more uncertainty in testing, supplementation, and utilization.

Even with my established patients who do their best to follow the Protocol, I frequently find insufficient absorption of vitamins and minerals. We can address this issue, but helping people effectively absorb nutrients is more difficult than people realize. The main factors involve clearing intestinal infection and strengthening stomach acid so a patient can absorb a useful form of zinc. Stressed adrenals and pancreas elevate cortisol, activate the sympathetic nervous system, push fight-or-flight, and weaken stomach acid, so addressing these components is often essential to vitamin and mineral absorption.

Finding supplements free of both problematic chemicals and food allergens that are absorbable when proper conditions are met is also a challenging piece. The ability to test people to supplements through sense of taste to confirm effectiveness within the body is powerful and illuminating. Unfortunately, most supplements test poorly.

It's surprising to discover that almost everyone tests poorly to a few plants often considered superfoods. When people taste blue-green algae/spirulina/chlorella, they no longer weaken to a reflex point that should weaken them. This doesn't necessarily mean blue-green algae is unhealthy, and many people claim to feel better when they take it, but it illustrates that blue-green algae interferes with the nervous system and is not a simple food. There may be a good reason to take it for the short term, but I see it as an interference to the Protocol as we work to establish clarity in the nervous system and address causative issues. A number of patients report that while blue-green algae was helpful when started, over time it caused symptoms.

Other supplements, herbs, or foods that create this same interference and of which I have mostly the same opinion are flax, ashwagandha, ginkgo biloba, valerian root, melatonin, reishi mushrooms, wormwood, and some of the other powerful medicinal herbs. They may be useful in controlling symptoms or compensating for some internal issue, and there may be a good reason to use them for the short term under certain conditions, but I don't see them address any causative issue, and they interfere with the nervous system. It seems especially strange that flax has this interfering factor. Possibly it's the processing or rancidity that I come up against, and perhaps it is a superfood when it's fresh or processed in a better way, but it doesn't test well with this method.

While pharmaceuticals always test poorly, of course sometimes they are helpful or lifesaving. Just because a drug, chemical, herb, or food tests poorly doesn't mean it should never be used. It means it somehow interferes with the nervous system and has associated side effects. As long as there is a good reason to use it, and the side effects are minimal or worth the risk, and there's no better way to address the issue at its cause, then it's great to have powerful herbs or pharmaceuticals to control symptoms. Unfortunately, mainstream and alternative medicine mostly treat symptoms rather than causes. While there are many reasonable justifications for this approach, it creates problems.

The following is a discussion of the basic supplements used to address the patterns of weakness and deficiency I find in most patients. Again, most people do not fully absorb these nutrients until multiple factors are addressed.

Ideally, patients come see me for guidance and feedback on the use of these supplements is ideal, but that may not be possible for everyone who reads this book. I plan to make some of these supplements available at theprotocolforhealth.com.

Calcium

Even the most basic of mineral deficiencies continue to baffle mainstream and alternative medicine. An example is the most apparent mineral deficiency that continues to become more and more problematic: calcium deficiency. Despite Americans being among the world leaders in dairy and calcium supplement consumption, we have the highest rate of osteoporosis in the world. Cow's milk doesn't appear to build strong bones, except with calves (baby cows). Every few years we're told a new story as to why no one really absorbs and utilizes calcium supplements or dietary calcium. Whether calcium should be combined with citrate, lactate, magnesium, vitamin K or "vitamin" D, the story keeps changing, and osteoporosis keeps getting worse. Part of the problem is that most calcium supplements are made from calcium carbonate also known as limestone—rocks—which are treated with chemicals. It may be that no matter how many chemicals are used, it's still hard to eat rocks. However, even when I recommend calcium supplements made from beet greens, they are poorly absorbed if people have weak stomach acid and intestinal infection.

One method of testing for calcium deficiency is a repeated muscle activation test that demonstrates that a calcium-deficient patient fatigues quickly. Calcium is needed for muscle contraction, so weight-bearing muscles are particularly prone to fatigue with its deficiency. After addressing stomach acid and intestinal infection, it can be demonstrated that only a quarter of the normal recommended daily dose of calcium (250 mg) clears this fatigue and assists with other symptoms. Many experts agree that 1000 milligrams or more of calcium per day is too much, but because it doesn't accomplish the desired effect, high doses are continued in the hope that some of it will be utilized and it won't cause kidney stones, calcification of arteries or other tissues, or contribute to heart disease.

Calcium deficiency is a huge issue, the worst aspect of which is fractures mostly in older people, but other symptoms less commonly identified and addressed exist: fatigue, cramping, low endurance, pain, and in children: poor growth, growing pains, and nightmares. Too often I hear of young people breaking bones from fairly minor accidents. This results from poor bone formation and possible calcium deficiency, inadequate absorption in general and/or elevated cortisol, which also contribute to poor bone growth.

One of the most closely associated and mis-diagnosed symptoms of calcium deficiency is plantar fasciitis, which is related to muscle fatigue. Muscle contraction requires adequate calcium. Without it, weight-bearing muscles quickly fatigue. The muscle tibialis posterior helps to hold up the main arch of the foot. When fatigued, the arch drops, stretching the plantar fascia. Combined with common inflammation, adrenal fatigue (that causes ligament laxity), and B12 deficiency (that causes ankle weakness), and the result is plantar fasciitis. Rather than look only at the foot and the usual mechanical and/or pharmaceutical solutions, this approach strengthens stomach acid, clears intestinal infection, reduces overall inflammation, and supplies food-source calcium to address the cause of the issue. General calcium deficiency helps explain our dependence on arch support inserts. While arch supports, anti-pronation shoes, slightly elevated heels, and spongy soles help people compensate for common weakness and deficiency, we were designed to walk barefoot. It's possible to approximate that by addressing the internal issues and with flat shoes with no arch support or spongy cushion.

I have—or had—flat feet. To try to control pain in my feet, knees, and spine, I wore three-hundred-dollar orthotics and a heel lift in one shoe from my early teens until my thirties. After addressing the causes of the issue, I now wear thin, flat shoes, and I can stand on concrete all day or chase my kids all over an amusement park without pain.

I recommend a calcium supplement made from beet greens that, for most adults, is best kept to only a quarter of the RDA, or 250 milligrams a day. Once people can absorb more effectively, adequate calcium can be supplied by eating the equivalent of a cup or more per day of cooked, calcium-rich greens, such as beet greens or kale. It seems easier to me to take the supplement than to eat that many greens on a daily basis, but I keep trying to eat more greens, as the whole plant and additional fiber are certainly beneficial.

Magnesium

Magnesium deficiency is apparent with muscle testing in relation to the heart. With this deficiency a previously strong indicator muscle weakens to two reflex points on the upper chest, at the second intercostal spaces, and the subscapularis muscles of the rotator cuff (Figure 10 below) will also be weak. The weaknesses are usually only apparent when a technique is added to stress-test

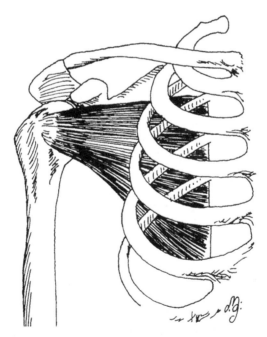

10. Subscapularis.
From the underside of the scapula to the front of the shoulder.

these reflexes. I find this deficiency in almost all of my patients, and it's rarely addressed with the diet. A cup a day of cooked greens may be adequate when combined with strong digestion. Between the calcium supplement I recommend and a couple of capsules of magnesium lactate (not a dairy product), most of my patients take a little less than 200 milligrams per day. With the Protocol in place, this quantity works well, but sometimes we increase the dose if constipation, muscle cramps, or difficulty falling asleep persist. Too much magnesium causes diarrhea for most people. Testing patients to supplements they were taking previously confirms that most react negatively to most magnesium supplements. This is likely due to the presence of synthetic components, citrate, or magnesium citrate, which are usually made from GMO corn.

B12 / B Complex / Iron

B12, B Complex, folate, and iron are in a supplement taken by most of my patients. Most B vitamin supplements people bring for testing test poorly. With muscle testing we determine if a supplement or food works or interferes with the nervous system. Often, supplements contain derivatives of corn, dairy, soy, or gluten, and if a person tests poorly to those foods, they usually test poorly to a supplement derived from them. Sometimes people test poorly to a supplement because of a powerful herb or chemical it contains. Even if a supplement tests well, it may not produce the desired results. Follow-up testing and a patient's symptoms make this apparent.

B complex and iron have many important functions in the body and are essential for building blood, transporting oxygen, sustaining health of the nervous system, and supporting stress management and memory. Compromised function in any of these systems has the potential to affect any condition of the body. People who repeatedly sprain ankles, or have chronic ankle or foot injuries, often improve when they can effectively absorb B12 because its deficiency causes weakness of the tibialis longus muscle of the lower leg (Figure 11 below). While red meat is considered a good source of B12, I find this weakness and deficiency in most of my patients, even those with strong stomach acid, without intestinal infection, and who eat red meat frequently. Therefore, I recommend this supplement for almost all of my patients.

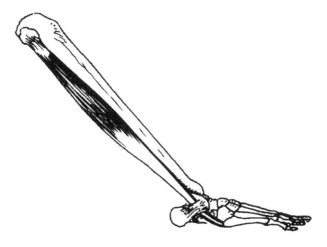

11. Fibularis Longus.
From the outside of the calf to the underside of the base of the big toe.

B12 is known to be difficult for many people to absorb. While genetics is increasingly blamed for this issue, the deficiency can usually be addressed if digestion is cleared and a quality supplement is used. Medical recognition of poor absorption has given rise to the idea of sublingual B12 or injections at a substantial price and with some risk. Both treatments highlight that the optimal system for vitamin and mineral absorption—our own digestion—isn't working.

Major and Trace Minerals

For full-spectrum minerals I use a supplement made from kelp. It supplies iodine and potassium and a variety of naturally occurring trace minerals. With a multimineral, it seems especially important that a supplement is plant-based. Ocean plants like kelp have the best chance of containing adequate iodine and all of the trace minerals needed because the ocean contains all minerals in their dissolved states. Minerals incorporated in a plant can be absorbed as food, unlike most supplements that contain ionic minerals, chemically processed minerals, or dissolved rocks. While it would be preferable to have kelp from a perfect ocean, that isn't available. Some forms of certified organic kelp test poorly and cause negative symptoms, suggesting the presence of food irritants or synthetic chemicals. Wild kelp from a reputable source used in a body capable of eliminating toxins is the best option I've found. There are many different minerals needed in the body, but the understanding of them remains limited, and some minerals have undetermined importance or are undefined as to whether or not they are essential. An ocean plant source enables us to trust nature rather than a chemist to provide what is needed. Dissolved rocks and supplements synthesized in a laboratory rarely test well or create the results possible with a food-based mineral.

Minerals extracted from ancient soils, sometimes called fulvic acid, have gained popularity in some health circles, and while I like the idea of using an ancient, unpolluted source, the supplement forms I've tested didn't test well. Also popular in alternative medicine is high doses of iodine, but as I said in my discussion of soy, this is unnecessary if soy is reduced or eliminated from the diet.

Minerals are needed for enzymes and other proteins and functions in the body; they're often deficient in our foods, and chronic intestinal infection and weak stomach acid interfere with their absorption. Mineral deficiency is associated with issues such as anxiety, panic attacks, heart arrhythmias, leg cramps, restless legs, and issues with skin, hair, nails, eyes, etcetera.

Because iodine deficiency stresses the thyroid, it weakens the thyroid-related muscle, the teres minor of the rotator cuff (Figure 5 page 92). This can cause pain, weakness, and instability of the shoulder, as well as nerve pain or issues down the arms and to the hands.

Using full-spectrum, food-source minerals combined with the other major and trace minerals (calcium, magnesium, iron, and zinc) also helps the body clear unwanted heavy metals or prevents them from binding in the body in the first place. This combined with the aspects of the Protocol for clearing intestines, liver, gallbladder, and kidneys effectively address the heavy metal poisoning I've seen among my patients.

Concentrated Raw Sesame Oil

One unusual supplement I use with most of my patients is concentrated raw sesame oil. This oil usually clears bilaterally weak gluteus maximus muscles (glutes), and/or sometimes gluteus medius or piriformis. The glutes have a neurologic association with male or female reproductive systems. Frequently, this oil clears complaints of hot flashes, erectile dysfunction, and low libido, and it often reduces hip or low back pain and joint stiffness while increasing energy. First clearing the liver and gallbladder enables a patient to clear excess estrogen or problematic estrogen-like chemicals and sets conditions for this supplement to impact hormones.

Sesame contains beneficial estrogen-like chemicals, which have been studied for therapeutic benefits but it remains poorly understood. The history of sesame oil goes back to ancient Egypt. It's also used in traditional Ayurvedic and other therapies. In looking for alternative sources, I haven't seen raw refrigerated sesame oil, or any other product, achieve the same results. It seems diet or other supplements could address this factor, but I haven't found a comparable solution. It may be that sesame oil is effective only if fresh or when sealed in capsules to prevent oxidation. It's easy from my perspective to identify the weakness created by the deficiency and observe increased strength and reduced symptoms when the supplement is taken. People with liver congestion, poor absorption, high insulin, or high cortisol are unlikely to experience much benefit from taking sesame oil.

Food-Source Vitamin A and D

It's difficult to find naturally occurring vitamin A without corn or soy-based preservatives. Few cod liver oil supplements are available in capsule form that don't contain synthetic vitamins A, E, or soy oil. Most of my patients take approximately 3000 to 4000 IU per day of food-source vitamin A. When the liver can effectively clear chemicals and excess hormones from the body, this dose is adequate. The greatest effect I've seen of vitamin A is the resolution of headaches and burning eyes when conditions are smokey in Northern California. This points to significant daily protection from dust, pollen, chemicals, and smoke provided by food-source vitamin A. Because of the support it offers to thin, sensitive skin and mucous membranes, it's useful with many sensitivities, and it often decreases bladder sensitivity, so patients are less likely to get up at night. Even the Mayo Clinic suggests that synthetic vitamin A, retinyl palmitate, may not be as effective an antioxidant as food-source vitamin A. Retinyl palmitate usually, or perhaps always, tests poorly.

Cod liver oil also contains naturally occurring D. While cod liver oil doesn't supply as high a dose as people usually take of synthetic D, I don't see any symptoms of deficiency in my patients with the dose I recommend. It seems everyone is pushing people to take "vitamin" D. Because we were designed to live in the sun but have moved indoors, this seems sensible. However, I have concerns about synthetic D. While it's said to reduce some symptoms, I've never seen the synthetic forms help any of my patients feel better, but to the contrary, I've seen it cause negative symptoms several times.

"Vitamin" D is used as a poison for rats and opossums and is dangerous to cats and dogs. For humans, it can cause high concentrations of blood calcium, which can cause calcification of soft tissues, heart, and kidneys, elevated blood pressure, and a variety of nasty symptoms. This is another good reason to use reasonable doses of food-based supplements and ensure a patient has strong digestion and absorption.

Biost and/or Rare Red Meat

With muscle testing, it becomes apparent that muscle injuries often fail to heal due to poor absorption of a component that is readily available in red meat prepared rare or medium rare. Many who consume pink red meat fail to benefit from this component due to weak stomach acid and intestinal infection. Once these factors are addressed, frequent consumption of pink red meat may adequately supply this nutrient, but most people don't eat red meat frequently enough.

To resolve muscle injuries that test well to this supplement, patients take three or four tablets twice a day for a couple weeks. For most patients, I recommend this supplement as part of the daily regimen to make muscle injuries less likely or to heal them quickly when they occur. Biost also helps with maintenance or building of muscle mass. I recommend it for patients who are over forty, athletes, or those who have been in car accidents or are planning to have surgery or major dental work. Biost can be helpful for anyone with issues of soft tissue failure or fractures, such as hernias, ruptured tendons or discs, blood vessel problems, gum disease, osteoporosis, etcetera.

Observing the rapid resolution of new or longstanding muscle injuries with the absorption of this supplement is yet another confirmation of the importance of red meat in the diet. Biost is prepared at low temperature to preserve the available enzymes that are found in rare red meat. In-office testing to this supplement often yields dramatic increases in strength and reduction of pain.

ZINC AND BETAINE HYDROCHLORIDE

As said in the introduction, I find zinc deficiency to be the most common, most problematic deficiency that leads to most other deficiencies. It's one of the first components I check at the beginning of every patient visit. If a person is deficient in zinc—which is what I find with almost all new patients at the initial visit—I recommend an absorbable zinc supplement taken with betaine hydrochloride (HCl) to ensure its absorption. Zinc has been established as essential in the production of cerebrospinal fluid, which bathes and protects the brain and spinal cord. It's likely this role in the central nervous system that makes zinc a key to establishing clear and accurate muscle testing. Zinc is also needed for stomach acid production, but it's difficult to find much research on this topic as most research focuses on how to reduce stomach acid and almost never on how to produce or supplement it. With muscle testing and by observing the resolution of symptoms, it becomes apparent that until people can effectively absorb zinc, they usually don't adequately absorb other vitamins and minerals such as B12, calcium, iron, iodine, and other major and trace nutrients.

I recommend zinc at the first visit for almost all of my patients and suggest they take at least this supplement for life. When new patients are already taking zinc, it almost never appears they are adequately absorbing or utilizing it. Also, when patients switch to other brands of zinc or stop taking sufficient HCl with it, I rarely see them continue to absorb it. For my patients I recommend Zinc A.G. and HCl in the form of Metagest, both from the company Metagenics. Without betaine hydrochloride, even my established patients usually stop absorbing zinc, especially in a period of high stress, poor diet, or cold or flu. Inability to absorb zinc impairs stomach acid production, interferes with absorption of all other nutrients, and may allow intestinal infection to be reintroduced. Patients who continue to take absorbable zinc and betaine hydrochloride rarely return with intestinal infection. Fairly often a patient comes in whom I haven't seen for some time, and they say, "Everything was great for a couple years, but it seems like all my symptoms have come back." This is likely when people have stopped taking zinc and HCl or switched brands or gone through exceptional stress or poor diet without increasing the HCL.

It may be that people commonly absorb zinc supplements, but without adequate stomach acid, it isn't in a form they can fully utilize. My testing identifies whether or not there is adequate absorption of *usable* zinc and demonstrates how important this issue is and how rarely it's addressed. Zinc absorption isn't straightforward, and health often hinges upon it.

Zinc is perhaps harder to absorb than calcium, and it's essential for the production of stomach acid, which is essential for adequate absorption of zinc, calcium, and all other minerals and vitamins.

Stomach acid production is also our defense against food poisoning and chronic intestinal infection. The Center for Disease Control recognizes that taking drugs or antacids to suppress stomach acid production increases the risk for travelers' diarrhea.

While travelers' diarrhea affects up to 60 percent of those visiting the developing world, intestinal distress from exposure to bacteria, viruses, and protozoa is common in all countries, especially when eating out. Strong stomach acid is our defense against these foodborne pathogens that often cause chronic intestinal infection. On several occasions my established patients have related stories of being the only member of a travel group or dining party not sickened by a meal—a testament to their effective stomach acid.

Zinc is almost always one of the keys to eliminating heartburn and reflux—symptoms usually caused by weak stomach acid, not excess stomach acid. While this approach is contrary to most mainstream treatments for these symptoms, we can always clear normal heartburn and reflux by strengthening stomach acid and addressing the diet. While diet and exercise are contributing factors to these conditions, zinc deficiency is usually primary. Weak stomach acid allows food to sit, bubble, and ferment, but with strong stomach acid, food digests and quickly moves on. Food sitting in the stomach too long can cause heartburn, reflux, or nausea. This is illustrated by patients who before care threw up if they ate more than just a couple bites of food. Their condition quickly resolved (sometimes in less than a day) when we put the Protocol in place and the HCl for strengthening stomach acid in particular.

Before starting the Protocol, consuming red meat causes symptoms for some patients, such as heartburn, a feeling of heaviness, lack of digestion, or nausea. Some patients cite this for the reason they became vegetarian or why they think there's a problem with eating red meat. Difficulty digesting red meat has always resolved quickly for my patients when they implement zinc and HCl. With strong stomach acid, red meat becomes easy and comfortable to digest, and many patients start to crave it and discover it to be satisfying and energizing. While some studies suggest problems with eating red meat, these studies continue to be debunked, but with weak stomach acid and intestinal infection causing leaky gut, digesting protein can be problematic. Protein digestion requires stronger stomach acid than carbs and fat, and undigested proteins absorbed into the blood trigger an immune response and inflammation. It may be that consuming red meat can contribute to health issues, *if* we fail to resolve the digestive issues common to most people. Otherwise, the idea that red meat is unhealthy is easy to dismiss if you believe in evolution or creation and you trust that hunter-gatherers have been eating foods we were designed to eat since the beginning of time. Red meat is the original superfood.

Unfortunately, the normal solutions for heartburn and reflux, such as antacids, baking soda, acid blockers, and proton pump inhibitors make the underlying problem worse while they are suppressing symptoms. Neutralizing stomach acid decreases the ability to absorb all of our nutrients and decreases our defense against additional forms of intestinal infection or food poisoning. These conditions lead to the prescription of more pharmaceuticals. Pharmaceutical companies scare people into taking antacids with the threat of cancer of the esophagus if the problem isn't addressed, but most people do not realize these drugs lead to malabsorption and the possibility of food poisoning and weakened defenses against ingested pathogens.

I'm certainly not alone in recognizing the prevalence of weak stomach acid and recommending betaine hydrochloride as a solution for heartburn and reflux. But I haven't found others whose emphasis is the use of HCl for the absorption of zinc to produce our own stomach acid. It's also important to identify the physical stresses that hinder this pathway—stress to the adrenals and pancreas. Many in the field of alternative medicine recommend HCl and strengthening stomach acid, and this was practiced by medical doctors as well up until about one hundred years ago when the approach switched to suppression of symptoms with chemicals and drugs.

It's interesting how the relief of symptoms from strengthening stomach acid with supplements or by drinking apple cider vinegar is obvious to so many but finding any mainstream medical mention of the idea is almost impossible. The few medical sources that do come up in search results say there are no studies on the topic and that apple cider vinegar might be dangerous. With an estimated 128,000 deaths per year in the U.S. from taking drugs as prescribed, we are cautioned by some of those who prescribe those meds that we should be afraid of apple cider vinegar? *It's fermented apples.* Not that I see apple cider vinegar as a full solution or that I recommend its use, but if it makes people feel better, it should be studied, and it's ironic at best that medical doctors warn people of its dangers. Death from pharmaceuticals often goes unidentified or unreported and the estimate does not include prescribing errors, overdose, and self-medication, so actual death by pharma could be two to four times that many every year, and it's rising. (Even back in 1998, the *Journal of the American Medical Association* published a study that estimated the number to be 106,000.) Again, this isn't about dismissing modern medicine but reminding people that drugs are dangerous, their side effects are constantly downplayed, their benefits are constantly exaggerated, and simple solutions that haven't been studied are held up as being dangerous.

How far modern medicine is from the solution of strengthening stomach acid is illustrated by a study from 2016. The researchers embarked to test whether or not zinc could help patients with GERD (gastroesophageal reflux disease) who were already taking, and continued to take, proton pump inhibitors to suppress stomach acid. The idea behind this approach is based on the observation that stomach acid decreases temporarily, immediately after ingesting zinc. (This is likely the reason zinc taken without adequate protein can cause nausea.) The researchers were working under the belief that GERD is caused by too much stomach acid, but as previously mentioned, weak stomach acid causes food to sit without digesting and to bubble up into the esophagus. Their idea was to suppress stomach acid further by taking zinc concurrently with proton pump inhibitors in a manner that probably caused nausea for many of the study subjects. Participants ingested 50 milligrams of *pure zinc* per day—a dose that exceeds the maximum recommended level of a form of zinc that does not occur in nature. Pure zinc is used to coat or galvanize metal to prevent rust (or digestion). To make the zinc harder to absorb they could have coated it with stainless steel... The researchers did acknowledge that proton pump inhibitors interfere with the ability to absorb zinc. After a careful three-month experiment, they confidently came to an eight-word conclusion that "Zinc supplementation cannot improve the severity of GERD." Which is true—when you create some of the worst possible conditions for absorption.

To recap the importance of zinc: almost everyone is zinc deficient; zinc deficiency is being made worse by atmospheric changes and other issues; we need zinc for stomach acid production; with weak stomach acid we don't absorb nutrients very well, including zinc; with weak stomach acid, pathogens gain access to the intestines and further interfere with absorption of nutrients; most zinc supplements are not fully absorbable or usable, and even the best forms of zinc may not be absorbed until intestinal infection is cleared, which requires an enzyme protocol almost no one is talking about. It is a vicious cycle, but the cycle can be broken, and people can learn how to keep it from returning.

Once my patients have cleared intestinal infection and established that they benefit from HCl, I recommend taking one to three tablets or more of HCl with 40 milligrams of zinc and the rest of the supplements after a protein meal on a daily basis. If patients experience unusual, significant burning immediately after taking only one tablet of HCl, they may need to stop taking it while we determine if they have a stomach ulcer or some other serious issue. Those with elevated cortisol, who cannot completely follow the Protocol, or with certain other conditions, may need to take more HCl as long as it causes no discomfort. In a period of high stress, poor diet, or cold or flu, the dose should be increased by one to three tablets of HCl for a week or two, or until the situation has clearly improved. The other time to increase the HCl is with any symptoms of weak stomach acid or poor absorption. This includes symptoms like muscle cramps day or night, nausea after taking the supplements that I recommend, or any heartburn or reflux with a reasonable diet.

It's always unfortunate when one of my patients continues to suffer symptoms when the solution is literally within their grasp and is so instant and predictable. Recently, one of my most adherent patients/friends had been going through a very stressful period. At some point she told me that over the past couple months, soon after taking her supplements she was nauseous. I reminded her of the solution of increasing the HCl by two tablets. The next morning the nausea was gone. Over the next few days she felt significantly better as her absorption improved and she got more benefit from the supplements. If this can happen to someone who has carefully followed the Protocol for about a decade, referred nearly one hundred thirty people, and supports those people in following the Protocol, then you can see how easy it is to forget a key piece relating to stomach acid. How many new patients have said, "These pills are making me nauseous. That doc is crazy," and never came back?

Weak stomach acid, with or without symptoms, and all of the conditions that it leads to is likely the origin of most aches, pains, and disease, and is the most important factor that tends to recur with established patients.

My system, which builds on applied kinesiology, creates clear instant biofeedback, which makes it possible to untangle the issues of digestion and absorption and demonstrates the effectiveness of recommended solutions. The key foundation is addressing chronic intestinal infection and the weak stomach acid that causes it. Almost everyone in the U.S. and probably everywhere is dealing with this issue, and its resolution is essential in transforming the health of my patients. Implemented on a large scale, it's a step toward transforming our collective health.

Emerging Awareness of the Gut-Lung Axis

An abundance of studies over the last five years make strong connections between gut and lung health. Researchers are exploring links between gut flora and a wide variety of lung conditions with studies, such as *Emerging pathogenic links between microbiota and the gut-lung axis, Inflammatory bowel disease and risk of mortality in COPD*, and *Desired Turbulence? Gut-Lung Axis, Immunity, and Lung Cancer*. It has been established that bacteria from the intestine can colonize the lungs and vice versa, not only by aspiration but also through the lymphatic system. Dysbiosis is blamed for inflammation in the lungs, which allows blood serum proteins to escape into the lung alveoli (air pockets), decreasing function and immunity and creating favorable conditions for pathogens. This liquid serum filling the airspace in the lungs contributes to bronchitis and pneumonia. The products of opportunistic bacteria appear to damage sensitive lung tissue, causing malignant transformation that can lead to cancer. Significant improvements in the allopathic treatment of lung tumors were accomplished in some studies by adding probiotics to the treatment. While the exact role of dysbiosis in lung cancer hasn't been established, chronic inflammation is known to be a factor in the development of cancer and most disease processes.

Studies and treatments of dysbiosis of the gut-lung axis focus on adding or supporting specific strains of beneficial bacteria—often with complicated methods of delivery. My results in practice lead me to believe it's not about these types of additions, but primarily the *removal* of chronic intestinal infection with digestive enzymes that allows the natural flora to bounce back in the absence of the pathogen. It's not about balancing dysbiosis or building up gut and lung flora but simply clearing chronic intestinal infection and preventing its return.

Recurring bronchitis and pneumonia with the tendency for colds and flu to settle in the lungs are conditions that resolve with the Protocol. For many, it's a predictable pattern that their lungs are vulnerable and every year they experience significant lung congestion or infection. Often, people can trace the onset of this pattern to an episode of illness from international travel, food poisoning, or other sickness. Working with these patients while they are symptomatic, we see accelerated resolution, and in the years following, they are much less likely to have similar symptoms. Clearing chronic intestinal infection and preventing its return appears to be the main piece to reduce or stop recurring lung infections.

These types of lower respiratory infections are *the number one cause of death* in low-income countries and one of the main causes of death with COVID-19 internationally. The number two cause of death in low-income countries is diarrhea, which is also associated with zinc deficiency and various forms of intestinal infection. Infections of the gut-lung axis are a constant epidemic in the developing world, but now with COVID-19, we are seeing a virus settling in the lungs and exacerbating the underlying condition of inflammation, with the propensity to fill the lungs with fluid, possibly requiring artificial respirators to keep people alive. The time to clear chronic intestinal infection and the related lung weakness is before exposure to COVID-19, or the next inevitable pandemic, or before we are of an age more likely to succumb to pneumonia from influenza, which is the eighth leading cause of death for people sixty-five and over in the U.S. Unfortunately, influenza and pneumonia are the fifth leading cause of death of children aged one to nine and have increased significantly in the U.S. in the last fifteen years.

Again, I'm not wondering about these connections. When we clear chronic intestinal infection with twenty days of enzymes and strengthen stomach acid, recurring lung infections and bronchitis stop or become much less common, and people feel their lungs strengthen and become less sensitive.

Other chronic lung conditions driven by inflammation and chronic physical stress, but in a less immediate manner, include lung cancer and chronic lower respiratory diseases, C.O.P.D., and asthma. While smoking and persistent chemical exposure are known to be the main drivers, many people develop these conditions without those exposures. The presence of chronic intestinal infection is likely why some have a tendency to develop these conditions, and why even simple wood smoke and dust can become significant irritants or carcinogens.

While it is established that zinc is important to the immune system, useful for treating diarrhea, and that the deficiency is linked to a variety of lung diseases, which are also connected to the gut microbiome, my system reveals how these conditions are interconnected, and breaks the vicious cycle of the inability to utilize zinc causing, often unrecognized, chronic, recurring lung and intestinal infections.

CHAPTER 8

The Fifth Cause of Disease and the Unexpected Solution

Overconsumption of Carbohydrates

Most of us eat too much sugar. Unfortunately, many people who eat a "pretty good diet" don't realize that fruit, grain, legumes, potatoes, and even the most unprocessed forms of sugar are absorbed primarily as glucose or simple sugar. How much of these foods can be eaten without negative impacts on our health depends on many factors, but mild aerobic exercise like walking or slow running significantly increases our ability to consume and metabolize sugar with fewer symptoms (Chapter 9).

Most people are addicted to sugar. Even if their addiction comes in the form of whole wheat bread, oatmeal, brown rice, beans, or fruit, suddenly reducing carbohydrate intake (sugar and starch) causes withdrawal symptoms for many people, illustrating their dependence upon sugar. Because most people eat carbohydrates at most meals, pathways for converting fat to available blood sugar are usually not very effective. If carb intake is suddenly reduced, some initially experience a dramatic loss of energy, mental fog, or flu-like symptoms sometimes called Paleo Flu. Others may experience strong or irrational cravings and/or a great surge of energy that causes poor sleep for a few days.

Many will not even try to reduce their sugar intake. Sounds like addiction.

Before you run screaming for the exit, I'm not saying to eliminate all sugar all the time, but there are significant benefits to eliminating it for at least two to four weeks and then determining how much carbohydrate can be reintroduced to the diet without a relapse of symptoms. While guiding people through the process of reducing carbohydrate intake, it's important to meet people where they're at. Some people can just dive into the diet at the beginning of care, and others need to ease into it by addressing the other aspects of the Protocol first. As a patient starts to feel better and have more energy, they may find it easier to reduce their sugar intake. When the process is managed well, sugar reduction often causes an increase in energy, better sleep, improvements in skin conditions and acne, and reduced headaches, neck pain, bloating, colds, flu, and inflammation, which then often dramatically improves arthritis or other pains.

It can be difficult at first to determine which piece of the Protocol for Health is most responsible for decreasing symptoms. For example, a patient sometimes thinks it's the reduction of sugar intake that has alleviated arthritic hand pain, but they might not have seen any benefit to cutting carbs if they had not lowered cortisol and addressed leaky gut at the same time. Putting all the pieces together simultaneously or over the course of a few weeks ensures that whether it's a reaction to gluten, vitamin or mineral deficiency, blood sugar instability, or any of the other components, the patient can see for themselves that they gain control over their symptoms. Moving forward they determine, ideally with muscle testing feedback, which pieces are most connected to the resolution of their symptoms. Improving overall health by following the Protocol decreases sensitivity to those main triggers as they progress.

When it comes to sugar addicts, I'm a good example. I used to think I had a great capacity for eating sugar. Over a couple of days, I could eat two boxes' worth of brownies and still walk away (usually). I would go through five pounds of mandarins in two days and think it was good for me. I didn't know why I got sick four or five times a year and had arthritis in my hands, or why I had recurring neck and upper back pain (it's not about "sleeping wrong"). Two or three days after I cut out sugar for the first time, I had to take half the blankets off the bed as my metabolism increased, and over the next few weeks I watched my pain subside, and over time my colds and flu disappeared. When some people cut out carbs they say, "Oh, I don't even miss sugar." Well, I am not that guy. I would eat donuts every morning if I could, and I still try some version of that now and then. Recently, I stood at my fig tree and ate twenty or more large, perfect figs. I felt okay afterward even though I don't recommend that much sugar for my patients. However, when you don't have any symptoms and the rest of the Protocol is in place, and craving calls, you may sometimes be able to get away with that sort of indulgence. On the other hand, another time I ran that experiment at our local gourmet cake shop. First, I had a serious piece of cake, and then I bought some cream puffs and macaroons to take to a friend. But I couldn't let her eat by herself. After that I was in a crappy mood for a couple days, and my digestion was off, but at first it seemed worth it.

With my system of manual muscle testing it's obvious when a person is consistently overconsuming sugar and starch, or exercising too hard, or not getting adequate mild aerobic exercise, or some combination of these three conditions—each presents as stressed pancreas with associated weak latissimus dorsi muscles (lats) (Figure 12 page 153). Weakness of the lats is another cause of tension in the opposing upper trapezii muscles of the neck and upper back (Figure 2 page 27). With testing we can determine a healthy balance between carb intake and type and duration of exercise. Pancreas and lats always strengthen when the balance is found. Whether the patient is a top athlete who is overtraining, a nurse who spends too much time on his feet but doesn't get aerobic exercise, or a little old lady who eats too many sweets, the weakness presents in the same way, and the solution decreases symptoms and improves performance.

Many of us find it difficult to moderate our sugar intake—because we love it so much! All the pieces I describe in this book facilitate finding a middle path or a sustainable route forward with our relationship to sugar. Again, the foundation starts with clearing intestinal infection. For many people, the bug living in their gut drives craving for sugar and/or starch. Sometimes people say, "I've tried, but I can't eliminate sugar from my diet." Eliminating sugar often becomes easier once patients go through the enzyme protocol so that intestinal infection stops driving sugar craving. Weightlifting or being on our feet all day, which both require a lot of muscle activity without sustained aerobic exercise, can both drive cravings for carbs. If mild aerobic exercise is added, this usually decreases sugar cravings and strengthens a person overall. Other pieces for moderating carb cravings are described in other sections.

When you give half an apple to a four-year-old child who doesn't normally eat that much sugar, it's easy to observe diminished mental clarity and unstable mood—not ideal conditions for learning or sane parenting. Half an apple contains about 10 grams of sugar, but a bowl of sugar-free cereal with milk has more like 40 or 50 grams of carbs that can only be absorbed as sugar. That would be about twice the daily intake of carbs for an active adult on a ketogenic diet, but that adult might weigh four times as much as the kid. What if that kid has the usual second bowl

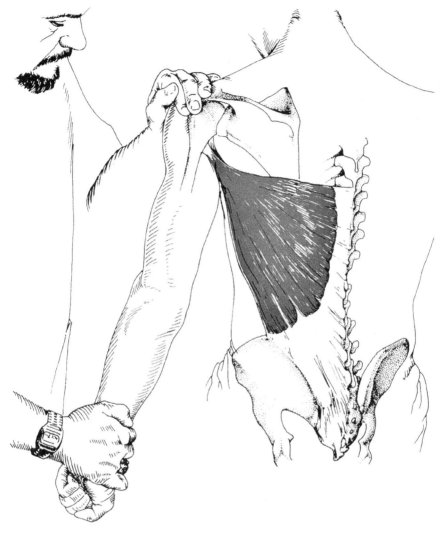

12. Latissimus Dorsi.
From the pelvis and spine to the front of the shoulder.

of cereal, or they regularly eat lucky-frosted-fruity-cocoa-junk? How could you treat the cause of ADHD without addressing the fact that this kid—and most kids, even those eating a "pretty good diet"—are saturated with sugar?

There are different ways to go about reducing carbohydrate intake and varying degrees of its importance and feasibility to different patients. For best results, at the beginning of care, I ask my patients to eliminate the vast majority of carbs and only include small amounts occasionally, such as a handful of blueberries, a little goat yogurt, or a half serving of starchy vegetables and/or to eat more of these if there is an immediate significant drop in energy from reducing carbs. This means encouraging people to eat meat, eggs, goat cheese, vegetables, and possibly some nuts. People may have to eat more fat, such as olive oil, butter, avocados, coconut oil, and fatty meats to sustain energy and possibly body weight. I mostly just encourage people to moderate their diet while keeping track of my guidelines, but some may need to measure quantities of their macronutrients and track their fat, protein, and carbs. There are many resources for how to carefully measure macronutrients and how to follow a low-carb Paleo or ketogenic (keto) diet. There are a variety of ways to test and to determine if you are in a state of ketosis, but that isn't important for most people, and the various forms of measurement have issues with accuracy, expense, and/or convenience. There are apps for tracking macronutrients and carbs in particular that may provide the structure some people need, but I find it tedious to measure and score all of my meals.

Many people quickly lose body fat on a low-carb diet and find it a satisfying way to eat, which helps them feel good and improves laboratory blood work. The satisfying nature of the diet is important, especially for those of us who have a hard time eating carbs in moderation. The reduction in cravings can come as a great relief and can help some with other addictions.

Some raise concerns about potential negative aspects of a low-carb diet for some sensitive groups because of possible stress to the liver or kidneys. This seems strange when you consider the foods people ate before the invention of agriculture—mostly meat and vegetables and not a lot of carbs. My testing identifies common stressors of liver and kidneys and effective solutions. Most people are dealing with a variety of issues that can make it challenging to transition off of carbs. By first clearing chronic intestinal infection, the related liver and gallbladder congestion, reducing inflammation, and addressing vitamin and mineral deficiencies, many potential obstacles are resolved. A low-carb or ketogenic diet is a useful tool for many, but it's sensible to first establish that the systems of the body are ready to process all of the chemicals that will be released from the potentially rapid breakdown of body fat.

Eating a simple, whole-foods, low-carb diet usually involves cooking for oneself, which is an obstacle for some. Cookbooks that focus on simple Paleo or ketogenic recipes, preparing larger quantities for leftovers, and other time-saving techniques, such as barbeques, slow cookers, and modern pressure cookers can make things easier. When buying prepared food or eating out, it's quite difficult to avoid the four food irritants, especially at corporate franchises primarily interested in selling the cheapest products—corn, dairy, soy, and wheat and meals with additives made from these subsidized foods. Independent restaurants, locally owned grocery stores, health food stores, and food delivery services specializing in Paleo, keto, farm-to-table, or slow foods are usually better options.

It's also important to recognize that eating carbs, while on a low-carb diet, causes craving for more carbs. This is why we sometimes feel like "there's nothing to eat," which is just code for "I've been eating too many carbohydrates, so now that's all I want." Some do okay if they avoid carbs for a day or two after indulging. In this way they avoid the sugar snowball effect. But for others, the snowball starts rolling with any carbs. With this type of addictive personality, a strict ketogenic diet is often the best bet. It's a way to go cold-turkey and break the addiction to carbs. I don't think the keto diet is necessary for everyone to sustain all the time, but when you're healing any issue, or trying to lose weight, or trying not to get sick, it can be an essential piece.

Avoiding Illness: Colds, Influenza, Viruses, Bacteria, Etcetera

The reduction in frequency, duration, and severity of colds and flu and other infections may be the most important reason for eating fewer carbohydrates. With the other pieces of the Protocol in place, and as long as there is adequate sleep, it becomes clear that carbs drive infections. Whether it's recurring bladder, ear, or sinus infections, strep throat, staph, the flu, or common cold, we consistently reduce or eliminate these issues but may see them return with excess carbs in the diet or possibly from just one overly indulgent meal. Again, this propensity for infection decreases over months or years as a person maintains the overall Protocol. There was a time when eating all of those figs would have likely made me sick, and if I did that after a few days of inadequate sleep, it probably still would.

Every aspect of the Protocol reduces the likelihood of infections. Chronic intestinal infection and leaky gut occupy the attention of the immune system and interfere with the ability to fight other infections. Problematic foods and the other factors that cause inflammation make infections more likely. Blood sugar instability and stressed heart (overtraining or not walking) elevate cortisol and tax the body, which suppresses the immune system. Sustained mild aerobic exercise plays a critical role in immunity. Walking thirty to forty minutes most days of the week combined with a low-carb diet are probably the simplest, most effective pieces for immunity that are available to almost everyone. Zinc is critical for immunity, and addressing the other common deficiencies strengthens the body overall, and strong stomach acid kills pathogens that might otherwise enter the intestines. When all of these conditions are addressed, patients can prevent infections or clear those that have been stuck in the body, such as infections of the sinuses, ears, bladder, boils, and cysts. On several occasions, the application of the Protocol made it possible for antibiotics to eliminate infections that had previously resisted antibiotics—a good example of the potential benefits of allopathy combined with this holistic protocol.

When you consider that the World Health Organization blames 18 percent of malaria deaths on zinc deficiency and that most people barely absorb or utilize zinc, the implications for the Protocol helping to fight infectious disease in general starts to paint a powerful picture. How about antibiotic-resistant superbugs, or the spread of tropical diseases with global warming, or Lyme disease, which is already an epidemic in the U.S. and resolves easily for some but is crippling for others? Fifty percent of people survive Ebola—why? As I write this, we are watching COVID-19 unfold. For a virus that primarily kills older people, why do young, seemingly healthy people sometimes die as well? I don't claim to have the answers to these questions, but my experiences with the forms of infections I have worked with leave me cautiously optimistic for the continued health of my patients and family.

Raising kids makes the role of sugar and its relation to illness particularly clear. If my kids get sick, it's nearly always after overindulgence in carbs. It's obvious even to our kids despite their bias for sugar. We do our best to be reasonable parents. We don't want to "deprive" our kids of the normal reasonable treats at birthdays, and holidays, and vacations, and grandparents, and friends' houses, and school snacks, and sports snacks, and free samples, etcetera; but what happens when you realize your society isn't reasonable? You cut most of the sugar out and then see what's actually reasonable. Or when they get sick, you consider what they have been eating for the last couple of days. Invariably, on the rare and mild occasions when we or our kids get sick, we have recently eaten more carbs than usual. Of course, there is more involved than just carbohydrate consumption, but if we know that viruses and bacteria thrive on sugar, wouldn't its reduction be a good place to start?

Applying the principles of Ancestral Health, we remember that before the invention of agriculture, less sugar would have been available during cold and flu season without ripe fruit. My patients and I find that we can eat significantly more sugar during the warm season without getting sick or experiencing other negative symptoms. Individual tolerance is variable with many factors involved, but adequate sustained, mild aerobic exercise is probably the most important piece. Personally, I do okay in the warm months with perhaps a couple pieces of fruit per day and occasional semi-healthy versions of junk food. For some, that is too much, and others can get away with more than that without stressing the pancreas, weakening the lats, and causing related symptoms. Some might choose to spend their limited carb budget on items such as potatoes, sweet potatoes, grains, or legumes if they tolerate those foods.

CHAPTER 9
The Sixth Cause of Disease and the Unexpected Solution

Lack of Mild Sustained Aerobic Exercise

The greatest source of stress to the body affecting most people in the U.S. is weakness of the heart and lungs—illustrated by the fact that heart disease is the number one killer. Certainly, diet and lifestyle contribute, but the fact that we used to walk for transportation and now we don't is likely the biggest problem. Most of us who aren't suffering the immediate effects of heart disease still have compromised health from a stressed cardiovascular system, which affects all aspects of our health.

Perhaps the simplest, most effective thing we can do for our health is walk. Since most of us in the U.S. drive cars, we only walk short distances. Carpenters, waiters, nurses, and others walk many miles per day, but only as short trips. This isn't the same as walking continuously for forty minutes, which gently elevates and sustains the heart rate. It's not about how many steps you take or how many miles you travel; it's about sustaining a gently elevated heart rate at a consistent pace. Some exercise is called "aerobics," but the emphasis is almost always on skeletal muscles more than the heart and lungs even if the activity elevates the heart rate. Many run, swim, or bike but fail to get the health benefits because they train too hard and at too high a heart rate. We've invented many fancy forms of exercise that don't look much like walking. While these forms of exercise can be beneficial, they can also be destructive if we don't have the heart and lungs needed to backup skeletal muscles. Because we often exercise too hard while suffering under the idea of no pain, no gain, many health issues and injuries are caused by modern exercise.

Carpenters, waiters, and nurses aren't generally known for their aerobic capacity or longevity, but the little old lady who takes a long walk daily keeps going and gets away with an imperfect diet. People who walk for transportation, a very small percentage of people in the U.S., have surprisingly few health issues. Backpacking enthusiasts tend to stay healthy as long as they keep walking. But in general, runners break down prematurely, those who play field sports have fairly short careers, and laborers have some of the highest rates of opioid overdose, largely because of physical stress and injuries that won't heal. These are generalizations, but these trends can be seen in life and research.

Creating an aerobic foundation by investing in six months of frequent, sustained, aerobic exercise is highly beneficial. Once this foundation is in place, introducing or reintroducing two or three days per week of anaerobic workout is a great way to proceed. Walking forty minutes *continuously* five or six days per week is a great way to create and maintain that foundation. Biking, swimming, rowing, or a machine that allows a similar repetitive motion also works to create this foundation as long as the heart rate is kept fairly low. Any form of exercise with a simple, repetitive motion and sustainable muscular effort that gently elevates and sustains the heart rate can create this foundation, but walking was our main form of exercise for a long time, so it is ideal. Walking on a treadmill or exercising on some other machine is fine, but without an audiobook, podcast, or screen it may become super boring. Swimming frequently for forty minutes, even in saltwater pools and particularly indoor pools, is a significant chemical exposure that creates health issues for sensitive individuals.

Exercise that focuses more on skeletal muscle, like weight-lifting, resistance training, lifting our own weight, or exercise that uses a series of different postures or movements to elevate the heart rate is beneficial *after* an aerobic foundation has been established.

A good test for evaluating whether or not a type of exercise works to create an aerobic foundation is to consider whether that one activity can be maintained for forty minutes without exhaustion or raising the heart rate too high. Push-ups can't be maintained for forty minutes, so while a person may benefit from that exercise after they've developed their aerobic foundation, it doesn't contribute to that foundation. Holding one's arms straight out for forty minutes can't be maintained, so a series of postures, including positions like that, is an anaerobic workout and focuses on skeletal muscles more than the heart and lungs, even if the series of postures elevates the heart rate.

What heart rate during exercise creates this aerobic foundation? Most formulas for target heart rate during exercise are too high or fail to account for various health factors. Dr. Phil Maffetone's guidelines work quite well. He's been working with athletes with heart rate monitors since the 1970s and has written several books on the topic. Many top athletes credit his guidance for developing their strength and health. The technique also applies to people trying to regain or maintain health. The basic formula is to keep the heart rate below one hundred eighty beats per minute, minus a person's age, with modifiers for state of health, years of training, and prescription drug use. This determines the maximum heart rate a person warms up to and cools down from during a forty-minute workout. While he recommends that number as a maximum, he points out the vast majority of the benefit can be achieved even if the heart rate is significantly lower. He also recommends a diet much lower in carbohydrates than most people follow.

Dr. Maffetone's Maximum Aerobic Function test (MAF) is a technique for monitoring one's progress and state of health. Essentially, a person should get faster at the same low heart rate over a period of months or years while initially creating this aerobic foundation. With this technique, athletes can eventually run quite fast at a relatively low heart rate, illustrating the improved strength and efficiency of their cardiovascular system in particular. In a race or athletic event, while skiing all day, or with an extra gnarly day of gardening and yard work, this translates into remarkable improvements in overall strength, stamina, and recovery time and reduced illness and injuries.

This training is ideally done with a quality heart rate monitor, but the simple version is to walk or do a similar sustained, mild, and repetitive exercise, making sure the heart rate stays fairly low while consuming minimal carbohydrates daily.

Most find that if they limit their exercise to this type of activity for four to six months, when they return to other sports, activities, or exercise their performance has dramatically improved. If they weren't previously exercising and are just working to regain their health, they find it a key to reducing inflammation, increasing energy, and improving blood work. Top athletes describe how foolish they feel training at very low intensity for four to six months with no speed or strength training but see their performance dramatically improve when they return to competition. They realize there's a better way to exercise than more-faster-longer. With the addition of this piece, regular people and top athletes see the full spectrum of health issues improve.

Applying this technique is challenging when people can't set aside their anaerobic exercise. Those whose professions include significant physical labor aren't likely to be able to take six months off for establishing an aerobic foundation. People who love their sports and/or whose fun and social life revolve around these activities are in a similar position. We try to find a middle ground. If they can reduce high-intensity and anaerobic exercise when possible and add forty-minute walks that help create the aerobic foundation with low-intensity effort, they find it's an essential piece of the Protocol. It can seem like a waste of time to walk when one is used to flying off jumps, cliffs, or waterfalls, or removing large trees all day, but the rewards become apparent in reduced symptoms, increased performance, and surprisingly increased strength.

One summer I had a ski instructor come to me who was recovering from a broken ankle. As soon as she was able, I suggested walking, working toward five or six days a week. Normally she prepared for ski season by running stairs and strength training. I recommended just walking and eating a reasonable amount of carbs and following the rest of the Protocol. She recovered quickly and also lost twenty-five pounds, an unexpected outcome that was previously impossible. When ski season started, her endurance and ability were significantly improved, and she had much less soreness after the first few days of skiing.

Applying this approach for a few months, most realize it works like some magic secret recipe, except it simply consists of walking and eating less sugar—exactly what people did before we invented agriculture and cars. When people try it, they see it's transformational. Unfortunately, it's contrary to most exercise classes, it takes diligence and time, and many forms of employment make it difficult to spend more time walking. People who walk or stand at work are constantly exercising skeletal muscle but not particularly the heart and lungs. This makes it more difficult to undertake this solution—they're already overtraining skeletal muscle—and it's less likely they'll want to walk for forty minutes after a day on their feet. If someone is sick and tired, they may not be able to take on walking, but without walking they may not be able to heal.

Emotional stress contributes as well, but when the physical stresses are addressed, it becomes obvious that emotional stress exacerbates underlying issues but isn't the real cause of health problems. When the seven main causes of disease are cleared, patients confirm that symptoms previously triggered by emotional stress resolve.

Long before people are at risk of dying of heart disease, they suffer from elevated cortisol and symptoms of the physical stress of having adequate skeletal muscle while not having the heart and lungs to back it up. This contributes to all pain, inflammation, digestive issues, and disease. The heart is a muscle. We must use it as it was designed to be used or lose it—prematurely.

I give the following directions to new patients for guidance on mild sustained aerobic exercise:

EXERCISE GUIDELINES

For the first month or two of following the Protocol for Health, the most important aspect of exercise is that it is not an obstacle to healing. Most people who exercise, exercise too hard or anaerobically, which in the long run may stress the body, raise cortisol, and cause illness, injury, burnout, and increased fat storage. Any activity which raises the heart rate too high or which cannot be maintained for forty minutes is anaerobic and leads to overtraining if there is not a sufficient aerobic foundation. Even yoga and aerobics classes are usually anaerobic.

People were designed to walk, but now we drive cars. When we exercise at too high a heart rate or focus on strengthening muscles (whether they are biceps or the "core") rather than strengthening the heart, lungs, and vasculature, we take the body further out of balance. Exercising at a low heart rate, at a sustainable activity like walking, running, swimming, biking, or on a machine that simulates these activities creates an aerobic foundation. Once this foundation is in place and is maintained, strengthening muscles with anaerobic training can be accomplished without pushing the body out of balance.

If you don't currently exercise and you don't have much energy, you might wait until your energy comes up to start exercising, but you might just start walking (or doing a similar light activity) at an easy pace and find that it increases your energy.

If you already exercise, consider how it is working. If you have health problems (injuries or pain, weight you can't lose, multiple colds and flu, or systemic health problems), your exercise may be part of the problem. For the next two to four months, tone it down. Ideally, stop any weightlifting, sprinting, "pushing" or activities that can't be maintained for forty minutes. What yoga posture can you maintain for forty minutes? Not many. If you do yoga or similar activity, it should either be set aside for a couple of months or done at 50 percent effort with no strenuous postures. Try walking or slow running. When you go uphill, slow down a lot.

Monitoring your heart rate during consistent sustained exercise is the key to exercise success. This is best done with a heart rate monitor with a chest strap (other more convenient types of monitors may be accurate enough), but you can get an idea of your heart rate by stopping during exercise to take your pulse manually. If you are ready to focus your attention on sustainable exercise, then follow the guidelines below developed by Dr. Phil Maffetone and/or refer to his work in *The Big Book of Health and Fitness* or at his website, philmaffetone.com. His technique may be used for overall health and/or for maximizing athletic performance. Many top athletes credit him for how they went from burnout to world-class.

How to calculate your maximum aerobic heart rate.

- Start with 180 points.
- If you have health complaints, take prescription medication, or you have not been exercising or you have been exercising too hard (from the perspective of this technique), subtract 10 points or more.
- Also subtract your age.
- This gives your maximum aerobic heart rate.

For example, if you are 50 years old and have a health issue or take a pharmaceutical, your calculation is 180 minus 10 minus 50 equals 120.

This means that your heart rate or beats per minute (BPM) should not exceed 120 while you exercise aerobically. In this case a range of 110 to 120 is the ideal maximum, but most of the benefit can be achieved even at 20 to 30 BPM slower. If you work with the maximum numbers, the first quarter of your exercise time would be gradually increasing to that number, and the last quarter would be gradually bringing your heart rate down.

Exercise like this for 30 to 40 minutes, three to six times a week depending on your condition. You may need to check with your medical doctor if you have a health condition. Eventually you might increase your maximum heart rate by 5 to 15 BPM or more, but plan on working at this rate for at least a couple of months. While it will probably seem too slow at first, give it a good try. You will get faster at the same low heart rate. For a thorough discussion of this topic refer to Dr. Maffetone's books or website. It makes sense and it works.

CHAPTER 10
The Seventh Cause of Disease and the Unexpected Solution

Unresolved Muscle Injuries or One-Sided Pain

As all of the factors in the previous six chapters are addressed, most patterns of weakness and tension, as well as deficiencies and inflammation, resolve with associated improvements in the absorption of nutrients, energy levels, sleep, and the immune system. Under these conditions many unresolved muscle or joint injuries spontaneously heal. However, some injuries and/or pain require extra attention and may need to be addressed more directly.

This technique of muscle testing can identify if an injury is present in one of the major muscles that cross the larger joints of the body or regions of the spine. Weakness from an old sprain or muscle strain is usually only on one side of the body and is usually opposite the side of pain. Once the injured muscle is identified, we determine if the solution is myofascial muscle work (usually rubbing at the attachment points), a nutritional factor that needs to be addressed (an enzyme found in red meat), or a technique of holding points for about twenty seconds (Chapter 11). These solutions work quickly and easily when the other pieces of the Protocol are in place but are unlikely to achieve lasting results without them. The solutions in Chapters 4 through 9 resolve systemic issues that cause specific patterns of muscle weakness, opposing tension, elevated cortisol, inflammation, and poor absorption of nutrients—poor conditions for healing. The more these factors are cleared first, the easier it is to resolve muscle injuries.

Neck and Upper Back Pain

Whiplash injuries provide an example of the process of clearing muscle injuries and pain. Most commonly these injuries are caused by rear-end car accidents. When hit from behind, it's the two prominent muscles at the front of the neck, the sternocleidomastoids or SCMs that catch the head as it's thrown back relative to the torso (Figure 13 next page). Pain and tissue injury is initially in the SCMs, but a few days later pain usually moves to the back of the neck or upper back, the upper trapezii (Figure 2 page 27) and/or rhomboids between the scapulae. These patients may come in a few days after the accident or possibly decades later with unresolved pain. While the pain is located in the upper traps, it's primarily the weak opposing SCMs that cause neck and upper back tension and prevent healing. The sternal head of the pectoralis major muscles of the chest (Figure 1 page 26) and the latissimi dorsi of the back (Figure 12 page 153) also oppose the upper traps, and their weakness usually complicates the injury. Most people have weak pectoralis sternal muscles because of liver congestion and intestinal infection. Clearing this reduces tension and inflammation and improves the absorption of nutrients to aid healing. Most have weak lats from pancreatic stress from overconsumption of carbs and/or lack of sustained walking. Consistent walking and a low-carb diet reduce tension, insulin, and cortisol and improve healing. Most people have upper back tension or pain due in part to stressed liver and pancreas. When there's a sprain or strain on top of that pattern of muscle imbalance, it's difficult to heal, even with the best-known therapies. When the pecs and lats have strengthened, it's much easier to identify and clear an injured SCM. The injury is cleared by rubbing the attachment points of the muscle for a couple of minutes, or sometimes the muscle weakness temporarily clears when the patient tastes a supplement made from red meat prepared at low temperature. In this situation the muscle weakness clears within a week of starting this supplement or from eating *and absorbing* an adequate amount of red meat prepared rare or medium rare so the enzymes needed for healing are intact.

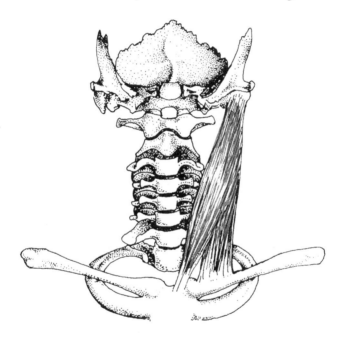

*13. Sternocleidomastoid.
From the sternum and clavicle to behind the ear.*

This approach reduces an injury to its key components, each of which has related muscle weaknesses and associated reflex points that can be tested against particular therapies that yield instantaneous feedback. In this manner we clear injuries that haven't healed over the course of multiple decades or from a week ago. Sprains and strains to areas of the spine, torso, and out to the hands and feet can be cleared with this process.

In some situations, neck and upper back pain is complicated by sensitivity to tree nuts causing weakness of the anterior scalene muscles of the neck. This issue is discussed in Tree Nut Sensitivities, Chapter 5 page 102.

Shoulder Joint/Rotator Cuff Issues

For about twelve years, I organized my life around whitewater kayaking. I especially enjoyed traveling, campfires on multi-day High Sierra trips, rivers in flood stage, and the eclectic kayak community. I'm glad most of us survived. Shoulder injuries are common in that sport. When kayakers come to me with shoulder injuries, the Protocol enables excellent results, so they can continue to huck themselves off waterfalls if that seems sensible to them. It's hard to see those who would like to continue kayaking but are stuck in the mainstream medical model of treatment, which rarely yields a great outcome.

One kayaker particularly illustrates the process of my practice and is rewarding to work with, despite his sometimes-loud grumbling. While I appreciate his skepticism, we spend too much time arguing about my suggestions, and he's literally cursed at me as I demonstrated his sensitivity to gluten. But in the end, he's willing to run the experiment to prove it to himself. He has described having shoulder pain and limited function a few different times for a few months that quickly resolved after a couple of visits. All is well until the next time he tries to chew gum (which usually contains corn, soy, and sketchy chemicals) and run waterfalls at the same time. His fitness is inspirational, and his athleticism is persistent as long as he's more careful than he was in his thirties and forties.

Shoulders are complicated not only because they're shallow sockets depending on the four muscles of the rotator cuff for stability, but because of multiple associations between shoulder muscles and a variety of organs and glands that are usually stressed because of how we live. The pecs and lats are the biggest muscles of the shoulder and are usually weak as described (Figures 1 and 12, pages 26 and 153). Of the four muscles of the rotator cuff, three are usually weak: the teres minor because of stressed thyroid from eating soy and/or lack of iodine; the supraspinatus because of stressed pituitary from corn sensitivity; and the subscapularis because of stressed heart from magnesium deficiency (Figures 5, 6, and 10 respectively, pages 92, 96 and 131). Considering most people with health issues have all five of these weaknesses, one starts to understand the prevalence of shoulder injuries and the challenge in healing. With these weaknesses, there is opposing tension, poor nutrient absorption, hormone and glandular issues, and elevated cortisol and inflammation.

I work with a pro downhill mountain bike racer who was repeatedly dislocating his shoulders from spectacular crashes or sometimes just from hitting a bump too hard. After we addressed the factors in the previous paragraph, his shoulders stabilized, and the dislocations stopped—while he maintained the diet.

In some situations, shoulder joint/rotator cuff issues are complicated by sensitivity to tree nuts causing weakness of the anterior scalene muscles of the neck. This issue is discussed in Tree Nut Sensitivities, Chapter 5 page 102.

Low Back and Hip Pain

Low back and hip pain have the same or overlapping causes because the muscles of this area have overlapping functions. Muscles that cross the hip also function as low back stabilizers and are responsible for trunk flexion and extension. Frequently, major muscles of the hip and low back are weak because of associated organ or glandular issues.

The psoas major muscles are perhaps the most important and most commonly involved muscles relating to low back and hip pain (Figure 3 page 31). They attach at the groin to the upper femur, cross in front of the pelvis, and attach to the five lumbar vertebrae, the bottom thoracic vertebra, and the associated intervertebral discs. Most people have weak psoas muscles because of two main issues: intestinal infection and reaction to cow's milk proteins. Other components that may stress the kidneys and/or weaken the associated psoai are dehydration, vitamin A deficiency, muscle weakness caused by calcium deficiency, certain foot issues that weaken the psoai, and statin cholesterol drugs that are known to cause muscle weakness and loss of muscle mass.

Weak tensor fascia lata muscles, which cross the hip and knee, are usually involved in hip and low back pain as well (Figure 4 page 50). The TFLs are weak when chronic intestinal infection is present.

If the above issues aren't addressed, it's difficult or impossible to achieve good and lasting results with low back and hip pain. It may also be essential to clear adrenal fatigue that causes weakness of the gracilis and sartorius muscles that cross both the hip and the knee (Figures 7 and 8 page 109). Weakness of the glutes often contributes and can be cleared with concentrated sesame oil (Chapter 7). Stressed pancreas with associated weakness of the latissimi dorsi (which cross the low back and attach to the lumbar vertebrae, sacrum, and pelvis) can also contribute to low back pain (Figure 12 page 153). Corn frequently causes issues at L5 at the base of the spine. After addressing all of these, any remaining muscle injuries in the area of the hip or low back can be identified and cleared. This technique makes it possible to determine the factor needed to clear a residual injury.

While many factors are involved, with my system and a compliant patient, all of these components can be addressed in four or fewer weeks with four to six office visits. Almost always, chronic pain either goes away or is much improved within two months or less of starting the process. Intervertebral disc injuries or other damaged ligaments are typically expected to require up to six months to heal. Indeed, after we have put all the pieces together, we may have just started the clock on healing, and perhaps it will take six months for a full resolution, but most issues heal much more quickly. Of course, if a person only has occasional mild low back pain, it may not be worth it to them to invest the time, energy, and expense, unless they're especially proactive about their health or have other related issues that are more motivating, such as IBS, food allergies, etcetera. Conditions like cancer, bone infections, or some forms of nerve damage (from disc herniation or stenosis) may require co-management with the appropriate medical specialist, but these conditions aren't necessarily obstacles to reduction or elimination of pain.

For a small percentage of people with chronic low back pain, certain exercises can reduce symptoms. These exercises usually fall in the category of "core strengthening." This has become popular in various forms of exercise instruction. The psoas major muscles are perhaps more at our core than any other muscle. Most systems of martial arts and most field sports recognize that every action starts from this area between the hips. While core-strengthening exercises can help some people to compensate for neurologic inhibition of the psoai and TFLs, exercises don't clear this weakness; they just strengthen muscles around the weakness. Studies show core exercises combined with chiropractic adjustments is one of the most effective treatments for low back pain. Unfortunately, that isn't saying very much, as even the most evidence-based techniques have a low success rate. Clearing chronic intestinal infection and/or eliminating dairy products from the diet and following the rest of the Protocol consistently resolves low back pain with or without core strength exercises. Weakened core muscles, caused by the increased prevalence of intestinal infection in our population, explains part of the trend of core strength exercises—almost everyone has this weakness because almost everyone has intestinal infection.

It's quite likely that scoliosis or significant lateral curvature of the spine is also related to inhibited psoas muscles. Scoliosis is caused by muscle imbalance and instability. Because the psoai attach to L5 through T12, there is no major muscle more associated with the stability of the base of the spine. As with low back pain, not everyone with weak psoas muscles develops the condition, but could the condition develop without this common instability from inhibited psoai caused by chronic intestinal infection? I don't know, but since there is no known, reasonable, effective solution for stopping or preventing scoliosis, this solution should be explored as an early intervention in the progression of scoliosis.

HEADACHES, MIGRAINES, AND JAW, UPPER NECK, AND FACIAL PAIN

In the last six years, I haven't had a patient with these types of pain who followed the Protocol and had anything less than 90 percent improvement. With these issues, inflammation and the effects of the four common food irritants are usually central. Again, diet has variable results without the other aspects of this approach. Clearing intestinal infection is also essential because the related liver congestion, hormone imbalance, and chemically driven inflammation can't be effectively addressed without resolving the intestinal issues. Inflammation is strongly associated with headaches and migraines. Blood sugar instability and elevated cortisol contribute to inflammation and pain as well. The ability to fully absorb zinc is essential as it is needed to make cerebrospinal fluid, which relates to these issues. The same components of muscle injury I describe as relating to neck and upper back pain may also be involved because the SCMs and upper traps attach to the skull, and imbalance and tension contributes to symptoms. These components underlie a variety of issues in the neck and head.

While all of the factors above have the potential to address headaches, the greatest trigger I see is cow's milk proteins. Muscle weakness from reaction to milk protein, which I describe in the previous section on low back and hip pain, also causes tension at the base of the skull and upper neck, especially on the right side. Many people realize their headaches start from a knot at the base of the skull before spreading to other areas and that these headaches disappear when cow dairy is removed from the diet.

Muscle imbalance of the jaw (temporomandibular joint or TMJ) is frequently involved with pain, especially of the head and neck. Specific muscle work on the opening and closing muscles of the jaw can be very effective when building on the foundation the rest of the Protocol creates. Applied kinesiology teaches techniques for clearing TMJ muscle imbalance, but the approach can be simplified, and lasting results may require careful avoidance of corn and adequate absorption of zinc. Corn triggers an issue with the pituitary gland, which sits in the middle of the brain and regulates the glands of the body. Corn also causes a neurologic component related to the first cervical vertebra (C1) at the top of the neck that also affects the TMJ because of a muscle connecting from C1 to the TMJ. Corn is probably the biggest driver of TMJ dysfunction.

In some situations, pain in these areas is complicated by sensitivity to tree nuts causing weakness of the anterior scalene muscles of the neck. This issue is discussed in Tree Nut Sensitivities, Chapter 5 page 102.

CHAPTER 11
Clearing Interference Simplifies Care

A few years ago, I was introduced to a technique for clearing interference that relates to muscle testing and can also affect physical symptoms. I had a patient who was carefully following the Protocol, but due to a complicated condition, he was losing blood through the kidneys. His blood count was low enough that he was scheduled for a transfusion. The patient went to an acupuncturist who performed "energy work" mostly without needles, and a week later his blood count was much improved, blood loss was reduced, and the transfusion was avoided. This blood loss had been ongoing for quite a while, and I had exhausted my options, so despite my skepticism, it was clear the acupuncturist's work had made the difference. I called him to talk about our shared patient/client. The acupuncturist's name is Stephen Barr. Stephen was also quite struck by this particular case, as he said he was able to do in one session what normally would have taken multiple. From his perspective, the physical components had already been cleared with my guidance, and all that remained was energetic. Fortunately, at that time Stephen was teaching his technique, so I attended his weekend course. While I enjoyed the class and had some inspiring experiences there, I didn't think his technique would fit my system or that it would create objective changes in muscle strength. I was wrong.

It creates obvious changes, and now I screen for this component at every visit. I borrow a small but significant piece of Stephen's technique, and it streamlines my practice by clearing components that appear as noise or confusion in the nervous system so that we can focus on more concrete physical indicators. It often creates some physical changes as well and can be a component in achieving lasting results.

This technique of holding points, or energy work, is most impressive or surprising when it relates to addressing a muscle injury. For example, when clearing a shoulder injury, if I find a weak pectoralis muscle and I've ruled out myofascial muscle work and nutritional components, I test for this energetic component. If the indicator muscle strengthens, I hold these points for roughly twenty seconds and retest the pectoralis muscle. Frequently, the patient can then push with approximately ten times as much force, and the pain is either reduced or gone. Every time I see this, I'm astonished and have no explanation as to why it works or why it usually has lasting effects.

Sometimes this energetic component shows up in relation to an internal issue or a part of the spine a chiropractor might adjust, or an applied kinesiology doctor might give some nutritional supplement, or an acupuncturist might clear with needles or herbs. Clearing this component by holding points enables us to remove noise or neurologic interference and see what concrete physical issues we might need to address. This also means fewer supplements are needed in practice than before because if an organ or glandular issue clears by simply holding points, we determine it's not a concrete physical issue requiring a nutritional solution. Clearing interference simplifies care.

An energetic component relating to an organ or gland causes associated muscles to weaken; therefore, muscles strengthen when we clear the internal issue by holding the points for the energetic component. This can be an important step for resolving muscle or joint pain.

Perhaps this energetic component should be considered the eighth piece of the Protocol. It has changed my practice significantly, and it sometimes creates distinct changes in my patients' conditions. While it may defy current scientific explanation, it creates obvious, objective changes in muscle strength.

Chapter 12

Glands and Hormones

Thyroid, Adrenals, Pituitary, Pancreas, Reproductive Systems/Sexual Function, and Problems with Blood Tests

Considering the complexity of endocrine issues, it seems impossible that any practitioner, up to the Mayo Clinic, could address the majority of causative issues regarding these systems. The interrelated factors and signals coming to and from the brain, the gut, and various glands combined with the impact of chemicals, illness, deficiencies, activity, and diet appear an impossible web of complexity. Add a variety of normal western medical laboratory tests, imaging, and biopsies that relate to particular aspects of the glandular system, not to mention many expensive, experimental, constantly changing tests used by functional and alternative medicine, and it's apparent that clear answers are unlikely. Even if a test result suggests you lack a hormone, neurotransmitter, chromium, or thiamine, how will you actually absorb and utilize it from a food or supplement? And if you repeat the test on a different day or with a different lab or technique, you are likely to receive a different answer. Modern medicine and laboratory testing struggle to achieve consistent results with *basic* vitamins and minerals let alone specialty supplements and synthetic hormones.

We must simplify by looking to foundational solutions like digestion, absorption, simple supplements, and diet rather than peripheral components or potentially dangerous drugs and therapies. But how to address the basics? Should we go vegan, vegetarian, Paleo, or carnivore? Low-carb or plant-based diet? Intermittent fasting or frequent protein? Aerobic or high-intensity exercise? Do we have too much stomach acid or not enough?

With clear feedback from the body, weaknesses become obvious as do the solutions. Yes, there is a need to proceed logically, and life-threatening disease should be ruled out. At the first visit with a new patient with a thyroid issue, do we start with specific micronutrients for the thyroid and the rest of the glandular system, or do we look at the big picture of whole-body health and make sure the patient can absorb their food and supplements? We start with digestion, absorption, and elimination, but since there is no consensus on what a person needs to absorb or eliminate and how to accomplish these goals, there's a foundational problem. However, my method makes it obvious which foods, supplements, and protocols work and which don't. A course of action becomes clear. Starting with the basics means emulating our ancestors before the invention of agriculture: they ate a low-carb Paleo diet, minimal amounts of corn and soy or other grains, and walked a lot.

By addressing digestion, absorption, elimination, and avoiding the common food allergens, most liver and kidney issues spontaneously resolve. We begin here because the liver and kidneys filter the blood and eliminate excess hormones and hormone-like chemicals, and these organs produce a variety of essential hormones as well. If excess or unneeded hormones and chemicals can't be cleared from the body, the cause of hormone imbalance can't be addressed.

The following is a list of glands and solutions to address their weaknesses. Weakness is indicated by any strong muscle that weakens when the patient touches a neurolymphatic reflex point, meridian alarm point, or pulse point relating to the gland. This weakness can be confirmed by testing muscles associated with that gland. When the gland is stressed, the muscles are weak on both sides of the body. The effectiveness of the following solutions depends on the extent to which the full Protocol is in place. The solutions may seem too simple, but for most glandular issues, the Protocol for Health achieves better results than anything I or my patients have seen in mainstream or alternative healthcare.

Thyroid

When a patient's thyroid tests weak, any previously strong muscle weakens when the patient touches the skin over the thyroid, on either side of the voice box or larynx. The teres minor muscle of the rotator cuff of the shoulder is also weak on both sides of the body, and the person may weaken to the triple heater acupuncture pulse point on the wrist when touched with light pressure. Each of these weaknesses temporarily clears when a person tastes a supplement that contains a natural form of iodine, such as that contained in kelp. The change in muscle strength is obvious and usually increases severalfold in a relatively healthy individual. A patient with shoulder pain may instantly go from barely being able to push with a painful shoulder to pushing much harder with little or no pain. The weakness may clear to a variety of other supplements or even chemicals, so further tests, clinical experience, and possibly blood work assist in determining an effective solution. I look to the simplest solutions first. For example, while a whole glandular thyroid supplement might strengthen the apparent weakness and may help the issue, a simple form of food-source iodine seems a more foundational solution, which also clears the associated muscle weakness and related symptoms.

If a patient is already taking a kelp supplement, but the thyroid tests weak, and we have established that they adequately absorb zinc and other nutrients, it usually indicates they have consumed soy in the last few days. Many alternative health practitioners use unnecessarily high doses of iodine because of the interfering factor of soy and/or poor absorption. Soy seems to interfere with the ability of the thyroid to uptake iodine. All of my patients with laboratory-confirmed thyroid issues clearly react to soy. This reaction combined with insufficient food-source iodine may be the primary cause of thyroid disease, but other drivers of autoimmunity may be involved (next chapter). When these factors are addressed, muscle weakness and reflex points associated with the thyroid resolve, and if the thyroid gland wasn't previously destroyed by autoimmunity, radiation, or surgery, its function usually improves or normalizes with the full Protocol in place.

It may be impossible to resolve thyroid issues at a causative level without simultaneously addressing absorption, elimination, aerobic exercise, a good diet, reaction to soy, blood sugar instability, basic vitamin and mineral deficiencies as well as most of the main factors in hormone production and regulation. When all the pieces are brought together, consistent, excellent results are possible.

ADRENALS *(see also Chapter 6)*

Adrenal fatigue and cortisol issues are surprisingly easy to resolve. For the majority of patients, simply following the Blood Sugar Stability—Adrenal Support Guidelines (page 106) reduces or eliminates adrenal issues. I think this piece would stand on its own in research and practice, but it's rare I only help a person to address adrenals without other aspects of health.

Supporting the adrenals means addressing the main reason they produce or overproduce their primary product: cortisol. Cortisol's primary purpose is to raise blood sugar. Keeping blood sugar stable with frequent protein meals in the busy part of the day decreases our demand for cortisol. Reducing cortisol affects multiple aspects of health, including inflammation, wound and tissue healing, stress and weight management, energy, mood, sleep, joint pain, and knee pain in particular, but cortisol's impact on hormone regulation is particularly important. If we're overloaded with cortisol or can barely make it due to extended overtaxing of the adrenals, it's much more difficult for other hormones to effectively regulate the body. Trying to resolve the causes of bad periods, difficult menopause, or symptoms of low testosterone may be impossible without stabilizing blood sugar to lower cortisol or restore our ability to make it adequately. Since elevated cortisol contributes to inflammation and interferes with healing, every condition improves with its normalization—elevated cortisol contributes to heart disease, diabetes, and cancer as well as simple aches, pains, and eczema.

Almost everyone is affected by this issue. Considering how common it is to have caffeine on an empty stomach or to drink too much of it, or to fail to eat a real breakfast, or to go too long without eating protein or not to eat enough of it, we see that most people are in an elevated-cortisol pattern. Our society is too busy, too caffeinated, and too sugared up, and is running on fumes because of weak stomach acid, inadequate protein, elevated cortisol, and overtraining. Cortisol is called the hormone of stress, and emotional stress is associated with most health issues and with elevated cortisol. But emotional stress is just the icing on the cake. The cake itself is made of blood sugar instability and *physical* stress, which is driven by the seven main causes of disease. All of these components can suppress the appetite and make us crave only carbohydrates. It's why there's *always* room for dessert!

Pituitary

The corn section of Chapter 5 describes what I see as the primary driver of stress or weakness of the pituitary gland. With the main pieces of the Protocol in place, removing corn and all its derivatives from the diet and using corn-free personal care and household products usually clears pituitary weakness.

The pituitary gland sits in the bony sella turcica at the base of the brain and helps regulate all the glands of the body. It has a close, demonstrable association with the first cervical vertebra (C1) at the top of the spine, L5 at the base of the spine, the supraspinatus muscle of the shoulder, and the TMJ. A common reflex that indicates pituitary stress is weakness when the right eye is closed or covered. It's probably no coincidence that many people cannot close only the right eye.

I've seen the resolution of alarming premenopausal pelvic pain, elevated PSA and/or prostate pain, TMJ dysfunction and/or pain, facial tics, tennis elbow, double vision, and other issues clearly linked to corn. Mental conditions like ADD, ADHD, depression, anxiety, and bipolar disorder usually improve with the elimination of corn. Most of my patients confirm feeling better overall without corn. Because mental fog is a common symptom of corn exposure and most of us are constantly exposed to corn, people sometimes find it difficult to connect corn consumption with symptoms.

With corn as an ingredient in most supplements, pharmaceuticals, prepared foods, bottled juice, preserved fruit and vegetables, toothpaste, deodorant, soap, etcetera, and given the impact on the endocrine system, the brain, and a variety of physical symptoms, reaction to this food is a huge, complicated issue. While it's usually sketchy synthetic chemicals that earn the title of endocrine disruptor, corn may be king in that court with soy close behind.

Pancreas

Weak muscles and reflex points associated with the pancreas are due to one or more of three conditions: overconsumption of sugar and starch, exercising too hard/anaerobically, or insufficient aerobic exercise (Chapters 8 and 9). The weak latissimus dorsi associated with this condition often contribute to neck and back pain. Resolving pancreatic stress is a factor in reducing bacterial infections, viruses, and colds and flu. If the pancreas must constantly produce insulin because of overconsumption of carbs, other aspects of pancreatic function are likely depressed, and digestion and hormones in general are more difficult to manage. When overloaded with insulin, small amounts of other hormones may be unable to effectively regulate the body.

Studies that suggest long-term health benefits from a high-carb diet of grain and legumes are studies of people who walk for transportation. Populations that consistently walk effectively clear sugar from the blood and increase sugar metabolism with less negative health impact. So maybe we can eat a ton of sugar, if we get rid of our cars.

Adequate, sustained, aerobic exercise is essential for tolerating a reasonable amount of carbs. It's how we lived before we invented agriculture—low carb and lots of walking. When this piece isn't in place, the pancreas is stressed by even a fairly low-carbohydrate diet. Without exercise or with too much anaerobic exercise the pancreas is stressed. People who run too fast, wait tables, work construction, lift weights, do Pilates, or vigorous yoga without adequate, sustained walking or other low-intensity aerobic exercises usually have weak lats and poor sugar tolerance. I was shocked when I stopped teaching and practicing strenuous yoga (which I taught for many years and had traveled a long way to learn), reduced my carbs, and started walking regularly or slow running: my chronic neck pain, back pain, and frequent colds and flu disappeared. I still think yoga is highly beneficial, but consistent walking and the Protocol create conditions in the body to either get more benefit from yoga or to achieve sustainable health without it. I certainly understand when patients are upset by the idea of temporarily stopping strenuous exercise they enjoy, but most confirm that it contributes to symptoms. Investing in an aerobic foundation is part of strengthening the pancreas, heart, and lungs, improving sugar tolerance, and eventually creates much better performance under strenuous conditions.

If the pancreas becomes exhausted from constant insulin production and/or insulin resistance has developed so we can't effectively move sugar from the blood to the tissues, blood sugar levels become too high and we're diagnosed with type 2 diabetes. The known causes of diabetes are elevated cortisol, inflammation, poor diet, and lack of exercise. Additional risk factors include high blood pressure, abnormal cholesterol levels, and a history of heart disease and stroke. These pieces are lumped together as metabolic syndrome. Recent studies show a link between gut microbiota and diabetes and obesity, which supports my model of chronic intestinal infection driving inflammation, leaky gut, liver congestion, hormone imbalance, and other factors that contribute to type 2 diabetes. We achieve great results with this condition; developing diabetes while following the Protocol would be extremely difficult if not impossible.

Far less common, type 1 diabetes is created by an autoimmune condition that destroys the ability of the pancreas to make insulin. The onset is usually in children or young adults. There has been some success in managing this condition with a low carb diet, and all of the pieces of the Protocol are helpful as they contribute to overall health. Because this protocol is effective with other autoimmune conditions, I'd like to implement it with children in the early stages of the disease when there's the possibility of halting or reversing the destruction of the insulin-producing cells of the pancreas. Considering the medical emergency and life upheaval this diagnosis creates for parents, it's a challenging time for additional supplements and dietary components. Parents may already have too much on their plate. Still, other than a diet lower in carbohydrates than the normal medical approach, I don't believe any aspect of this method is contrary to standard treatments. The Protocol is simply about diet, exercise, digestive enzymes, and mostly food-based, simple supplements.

Reproductive Systems/Sexual Function

In general, male and female hormone issues have the same underlying causes and respond well to the Protocol for Health. With the rest of the Protocol in place, it becomes apparent that concentrated raw sesame oil often has profound benefits for these systems (Chapter 7). Sesame oil clears common weaknesses of reflex points and muscles associated with reproductive systems and is therefore a component of the Protocol. With all of the other pieces in place, symptoms that often resolve with the use of sesame oil include hot flashes, erectile dysfunction, and hip and low back pain, but any sex hormone or glute strength-related symptom can be affected.

Female Hormone Issues and Dysmenorrhea

One of the most rewarding types of patients to work with are those with challenging menstrual periods. In most cases, by two to four months into the Protocol, the monthly cycle is reasonable and mild. I don't say this lightly. I can only imagine the experience of hormonally driven pain, moods, or other significant issues every month. We consistently clear these symptoms. The results illustrate the effectiveness of the Protocol for addressing the glandular system and balancing hormones.

Symptoms around the menstrual cycle or in menopause become clear indicators of the effective application of this system. The frequency and intensity of hot flashes effectively indicate whether a solution is in place and can help to expose previously unidentified irritants. This may reveal a patient's sensitivity to tree nuts or cane sugar or reactions to potential irritants such as fumes from a memory foam mattress or workplace chemical exposure. To set conditions for patients to clearly connect irritants with symptoms, people carefully follow the Protocol for at least a couple of months to establish a clear baseline where symptoms are less frequent and no longer seem random. Once the cause of symptoms can be seen, people can make informed choices about diet, exercise, etcetera, to control these symptoms.

While each of the components of the Protocol can be essential for achieving results, success particularly hangs on the importance of clearing chronic intestinal infection because of its effects on the liver and gallbladder. Clearing leaky gut means stopping the source of liver congestion. When liver function is improved, a person more effectively clears excess hormones or hormone-like chemicals, and the foundation is set for true hormone balancing.

The use of so-called bioidentical hormones, birth control pills, or other synthetic hormones can relieve mild to terrible symptoms, but unfortunately, they come with some risks and don't address underlying causes. Many women have bad reactions or significant side effects due to synthetic hormones. It's established that our own hormones out of balance can cause serious problems or disease, let alone adding chemicals on top of this imbalance. Safe options that allow the body to function as designed should be considered first. Because symptoms can be so terrible (pain, heavy bleeding, mood swings, serious mental health issues, etc.), anything that helps can literally be a lifesaver. However, when the underlying cause is addressed, better results can be achieved, and the solution *contributes* to a patient's overall strength and health rather than carrying the risk of serious side effects.

Birth control pills, other hormonal birth control, and non-hormone IUDs can play an essential role in women's choices, but their impact on health, athletic performance, and the risk of serious complications remain poorly understood and seriously lacking in quality, independent studies. The body's natural systems are too complicated to add synthetic hormones without adding the risk of serious side effects that are likely to be underreported, minimized, and understudied. How many women permanently lose their monthly cycle, the important long-term health benefits associated with it, and permanently lose the ability to become pregnant because of birth control? How many women die or have serious complications from blood clots and other factors because of synthetic hormones? It's not easy to get answers. Certainly, much more common are symptoms dismissed by others as inconvenient, but which greatly impact quality of life and mental health and for which there is even less available information. It may be it's simply the complexity of the systems involved that accounts for the lack of data in this area, but it's hard not to feel that the lack of research and tracking is related to women's issues in general and that it's contrary to the interests of the pharmaceutical industry to study and report side effects.

Helping patients transition from synthetic hormones to a better solution is usually comfortable and effective, and people are happier with the results. Because I can't make any recommendations around pharmaceuticals, patients should talk with their medical doctors about trying a reduced hormone dose at about one month into the Protocol because at that time the solution starts to address the underlying imbalance. If birth control is used to control negative symptoms, not pregnancy, a conversation with an M.D. may be required. If a patient doesn't reduce their synthetic hormones quickly enough, the pharmaceuticals that once helped control symptoms become the component that prevents the natural balancing of hormones. This transition in care can be tricky. Patients realize the chemical that was helping is now preventing a solution. Having an open-minded M.D. to guide the patient in slowly reducing the prescription over the course of a couple of months helps greatly, but this doesn't seem possible with birth control that likely can't be taken at a reduced dosage. With the full Protocol, the transition off of synthetics is usually comfortable. However, ingesting corn, soy, or other irritants can make the process variable, but it may demonstrate the effects of the irritants to the patient. Certainly, the process is less complicated if prescription drugs aren't involved in the first place.

This technique's consistent resolution of hormone-related symptoms puts me in a unique position to distinguish the side effects of birth control and added hormones from other hormone issues. It has become apparent to me and some of my patients that even copper IUDs, which don't deliver synthetic hormone, can have a profound effect on hormone-related symptoms. As with all invasive procedures and drugs, the risks versus benefits of any internal birth control or added hormones must be weighed, and the choice is personal, but it's easy to see that adding these components complicates my patients' health.

When the Protocol is applied to fertility, pregnancy, birth, and lactation, the results can seem like miracles. I don't claim to treat these conditions, but when patients remove the obstacles to natural hormonal controls, the body is much more likely to do what it was designed to do. It's rewarding to help pregnant women and new moms with their symptoms. Consistent, effective results are achieved with their low back pain, low energy, morning sickness, persistent nausea, lactation issues, and postpartum depression.

I worked with a couple who had tried many therapies and were about to spend twenty to sixty thousand dollars on in vitro fertilization (IVF). Four months into care they conceived. I have other couples who credit the Protocol for their pregnancies as well.

Birth stories of women in my care usually describe a relatively short labor without complications. For my wife and me, our first daughter was born five and a half hours after contractions started. Our second daughter was forty-eight minutes. Both were home births with no complications. Without the hormone/chemical overload common to most people, natural hormone controls are more effective at regulating processes of fertilization, pregnancy, birth, lactation, and postpartum recovery. It's amazing to see birth proceed unhindered.

Male Hormone Issues

Helping men with issues such as prostate, low testosterone, low libido, or erectile dysfunction is quite similar to working with women. While that may sound odd, hormone solutions are about removing obstacles to natural function so the body can do what it was designed to do. The foundation is to enable absorption and utilization of basic nutrients to fuel and maintain the body and eliminate chemicals and other components interfering with the glandular system. Making sure the liver clears excess estrogen-like chemicals may be the key to addressing a variety of symptoms caused by relatively low testosterone. Excessive cortisol in the body from blood sugar instability and lack of aerobic exercise can be the source of hormone insufficiency or imbalance. Corn and soy and their impact on the pituitary and thyroid are often critical components. Strengthening stomach acid to ensure the absorption of key nutrients can create profound changes within a week or two. Usually, a combination of these factors and other aspects of the Protocol work together to address male hormone issues.

A recent example involves a man in his sixties who's been in my practice for a few years but hadn't been in for several months. His libido and erectile function were low. In-office testing confirmed he had stopped fully absorbing zinc, so his stomach acid was weak, and he wasn't effectively absorbing the Basic 9 supplements. Zinc is also essential for prostate health. In looking further, his adrenals were stressed from neglecting blood sugar stability, as was the pancreas due to consuming too many beans with corn-free chips. Such factors elevate cortisol and insulin, suppress digestion, and make it harder to absorb zinc. At least he was walking consistently, avoiding the food irritants, and taking the basic supplements. I suggested he increase the betaine hydrochloride for a couple of weeks while he addressed his diet. When we followed up three weeks later, he had improved by 70 percent, but he was still eating too much carbohydrate. At the next follow-up visit and since then, he's happy with the results. He's proven to himself how important these factors are for feeling young.

Problems with Blood Tests

You've probably gathered I'm not overly impressed by many of the blood tests currently available. What about screening for disease, such as testing for elevated cholesterol, blood sugar, hormone levels, and other factors? Here again we see the limited ability of some lab tests to yield information relevant to the health of an individual. Problems arise from comparing test results to average test values that aren't necessarily relevant to patients whose diet, exercise, and nutrient absorption aren't average. It's not uncommon for patients who follow the Protocol to have slightly elevated total cholesterol but low triglycerides, low LDL cholesterol levels ("the bad type"), and a good ratio of HDL cholesterol to total cholesterol, which all indicate a supposedly low-risk category for heart disease. Some medical doctors still prescribe cholesterol meds for this patient or resist lowering or stopping the med when blood work improves. However, most studies are funded by the pharmaceutical industry and many people with high cholesterol do not suffer from heart disease, and many people with low cholesterol suffer from heart disease, so it's hard to know how much faith to put into these numbers. Burning fat more efficiently, because of consistent low-carb intake, helps patients clear excess cholesterol from the blood. It's particularly important that these people fast before a cholesterol test, so their base levels of cholesterol are measured rather than the contents of their last meal.

Fasting blood glucose tests may also present a problem for my patients because efficient fat conversion to available blood sugar may keep blood glucose levels slightly elevated during fasting. This indicates a metabolism that sustains blood sugar levels better than most, not overconsumption of carbs and decreased ability to metabolize sugar. In this case the slightly elevated blood sugar helps fuel the body and keep energy levels stable, but it can lead an M.D. to think diabetes is developing or that a patient shouldn't decrease their diabetes drugs because the blood sugar is higher than the level considered normal. When people don't eat a normal diet or suffer from the normal causes of disease, does it make sense to compare their lab work to a normal population? Probably not, but it's unlikely there will be a definitive study for this population any time soon.

On the other hand, there are lab tests that demonstrate the normalizing effects of the overall Protocol. Cholesterol and blood sugar levels far out of normal range improve significantly, as do numbers for blood clotting, PSA (prostate), thyroid, pituitary, hemoglobin, and a variety of hormone levels and inflammatory markers. I rarely order these blood tests, but when people are working with an M.D. and are tracking these numbers, we see improvements with these tests.

Sometimes people make the mistake of ordering blood work during the process of the twenty-day enzyme protocol. Here again we see the enzymes clearly affecting the liver and gallbladder as these people may show a temporary increase in liver enzymes, cholesterol, hormones, or inflammatory markers. This is simply a function of the enzymes clearing accumulated waste products and sludge that has been stuck in our most essential filter, the liver. This altered lab result highlights the efficacy of simple digestive enzymes. It also illustrates the reason patients sometimes need to slow or pause taking them. By two or three weeks after the enzymes, these numbers are back down or usually better than before. Having elevated liver enzymes is a non-specific condition usually monitored by medical doctors until it's bad enough to take multiple biopsies (pieces cut out of the liver) to check for cancer or other pathology. As long as immediate life-threatening issues have been ruled out, it's sensible to try a safe, simple protocol before the condition develops into the need for a potentially lethal biopsy.

Whether blood tests are related to cholesterol, blood sugar, thyroid, pituitary, or other systems, one simple test isn't enough to warrant starting a prescription medication. Other tests should be included for more information about the whole situation. Guidelines for drug prescription almost always state that solutions including diet, exercise, and lifestyle should be implemented before adding drugs to the body. Studies confirm that prescriptions usually lead to more prescriptions because of drug side effects and unresolved underlying issues. It's almost always easier to find an effective solution before starting a pharmaceutical, rather than figuring out how to get off of it later. Side effects of drugs are chronically down-played, underreported, unknown, or nearly impossible to connect to the drug. Too often, decades later, science finally realizes the negative impacts of controlling a symptom with a drug. Considering the difficulty of getting an answer about something as fundamental as a negative reaction to gluten, adding synthetic chemicals to the body seems an especially dangerous act of faith.

Chapter 13

Solving Difficult Issues

Weight Loss, Inability to Gain Weight, Blood Pressure, Autoimmunity, Rheumatoid Arthritis, MS, Fibromyalgia, Chronic Fatigue, Carpal Tunnel/Repetitive Stress Injury, Lyme Disease, Migraines, Narcolepsy, Insomnia, Addiction, Depression, Anxiety/Panic/Heartbeat Irregularities

As with all conditions, solutions to these issues include setting in motion the seven components of the Protocol for Health and clearing the obstacles to healing. Here are additional comments for these conditions.

Weight Loss

I won't bore you with the usual tirade about how we have a collective weight problem. Most pain and disease are usually blamed on excess body fat, at least when people are carrying extra weight. It's the classic doctor cop-out to tell a person their low back pain, sleep apnea, foot pain, etcetera won't resolve until they lose some weight. It's almost as cliché as telling a person to reduce their stress or that their symptoms are only in their head, and they'll have to take some not-so-groovy drugs. Sure, losing weight or the right pharmaceutical intervention can be a lifesaver and can reduce symptoms, but applying simple solutions that work usually resolves symptoms and contributes to health whether or not people lose the weight.

One excellent side effect of this process is the frequent "accidental" loss of unwanted weight while eating a satisfying diet without measuring portions. Even if it is a patient's goal, for the first two months of care, I encourage them not to focus on weight loss, and instead to establish health, energy, and the ability to walk consistently or perform a similar exercise. Sometimes people lose as much as fifteen pounds in the first two weeks of care, largely from the reduction of bloating, water retention, and inflammation. While this can be alarming to some, this type of weight loss is always beneficial, even if body fat was already low. Sometimes older people are concerned they will lose too much weight, or family or friends become concerned when they see their weight loss. Remember that maintaining muscle mass, not extra body fat, is the real indicator of health. To maintain muscle mass, I suggest my patients eat muscle—meat, or some other form of protein frequently—and eat enough fat to fuel the body and maybe a few carbs. If a patient feels they're getting too lean, they can increase fat intake and possibly protein as well. Good fat sources include nuts (if digestion is good), goat cheese, fatty meats, avocados, olive oil, butter, etcetera.

Weight loss is another example of a condition where any one of the seven factors can be an obstacle to achieving results. If weak stomach acid and/or intestinal infection is causing deficiencies, there may be constant hunger because the body is essentially starving for certain nutrients, driving overeating. Liver congestion from leaky gut or endocrine issues caused by food reactions or mineral deficiencies can cause hormone imbalance, making weight loss more difficult. Eating carbs prompts craving for more carbs, which often leads to overeating. Some find it nearly impossible to step away from carbs until intestinal infection is cleared. Blood sugar instability frequently causes people to overeat. Elevated cortisol is known to prevent weight loss. Cortisol is elevated by infrequent protein or exercising too hard or too anaerobically without an aerobic foundation. Some need anaerobic exercise to lose weight. Without an aerobic foundation like six months of walking, anaerobic exercise may work for a couple of months but is then likely to elevate cortisol, cause injury, illness, or burnout as the body becomes overly stressed from pushing skeletal muscle without having the heart and lungs to back it up.

For some, the seven solutions create conditions for steady weight loss until optimal weight is achieved without having to focus on weight loss. These patients are astonished as they have to keep buying smaller clothes.

Unfortunately, weight loss isn't that simple for everyone, but the Protocol clears obstacles and sets conditions that facilitate weight loss and the ability to keep it off. An individual may need to focus on the form of exercise, portion control, and/or careful measuring and tracking of macronutrients, even if those routes were previously unsuccessful. The process of weight loss becomes fundamentally different with the Protocol in place, but we may choose to carry some extra weight because of our love of food, or our unwillingness to exercise adequately. However, extra body fat is less likely to be an obstacle to health when inflammation decreases, symptoms resolve, and particular health markers improve, as chosen by you and/or your doctor.

Inability to Gain Weight

See Chapter 6: Appetite, Eating, and Absorption.

Blood Pressure

Abnormal blood pressure, whether it's too high or too low, can create a variety of negative symptoms, and high blood pressure increases the risk of heart disease, stroke, diabetes, kidney damage, blindness, and other issues. A recent study found that 18 percent of deaths include high blood pressure as a contributing factor. While genetics, eating meat, and salt are often blamed for high blood pressure, these factors don't prevent my patients from normalizing blood pressure to healthy levels. I don't think I've had an adherent patient in the last five or six years who couldn't get off of blood pressure meds and sustain healthy blood pressure.

Autoimmunity

Autoimmunity includes many different conditions, from well-known to obscure. The core of the issue is an immune system with an inappropriate reaction that becomes self-destructive. The cause is unknown and conventional drug treatments are poor and ultimately cause more symptoms or disease.

The model of chronic intestinal infection causing leaky gut, liver congestion, poor absorption, food sensitivities, and inflammation offers a probable explanation of autoimmunity. The immune system's constant battle with a pathogen living in the gut and the reaction to undigested food proteins entering the blood sets the stage. Inability to clear chemicals and excess hormones, vitamin and mineral deficiencies, inflammation, and glandular issues result. Elevated cortisol compromises the ability to heal damage caused by these issues. Resolving these issues always reduces autoimmunity.

Rheumatoid Arthritis

While rheumatoid arthritis is an autoimmune condition, it's like other forms of arthritis in that it comes down to joint inflammation. As the Protocol significantly reduces inflammation, joint pain improves, as does the overall ability to heal. With visible joint deformation, it's unlikely the deformity can be greatly reversed, but pain and progression can be reduced or eliminated.

Multiple Sclerosis (MS)

As an autoimmune condition of the central nervous system, drug treatments for multiple sclerosis are poor, and symptoms are complicated and often seem random. Reducing inflammation decreases the pressure of sclerotic lesions on nerves. Nerves are very sensitive to small amounts of pressure, so even a slight decrease in inflammation, and therefore pressure, can significantly improve a variety of symptoms. The Protocol always reduces inflammation significantly so that symptoms of MS either improve or resolve.

Fibromyalgia and Chronic Fatigue

Fibromyalgia and chronic fatigue are mostly driven by the interaction of chronic intestinal infection, reactions to common foods, inflammation, and symptoms of vitamin and mineral deficiency. Addressing these issues, people improve quickly.

I had a patient with fibromyalgia who, at the first follow-up appointment one week into care said, without humor, "Well, I almost didn't come back because I feel so much better, and I was afraid you might screw it up." It's a funny but sad comment because people are so certain there's no solution.

Carpal Tunnel and Repetitive Stress Injuries

Carpal tunnel syndrome generally remains poorly understood, frequently misdiagnosed, and ineffectively treated. I've had great success with many with this condition. There is a known association with carpal tunnel and hypothyroidism. I find soy is often the main driver of both. While soy isn't the only factor in carpal tunnel, I've seen cases where symptoms of full-on paralysis with compromised nerve conduction velocity disappeared with soy elimination.

Repetitive stress injury is sometimes considered the cause of carpal tunnel syndrome and other conditions. These injuries are associated with any repetitive activity involving work, sports, typing, texting, video games, etcetera. While these conditions have become normal, most of the time they make no sense. Typing or using a mouse, even for too many hours a day, should not cause injury. When we reduce inflammation and improve conditions so the body can heal, these issues resolve.

Lyme Disease

With an estimated three hundred thousand new cases of Lyme disease annually in the U.S. and an unfortunately large but debated percentage of those treated with antibiotics still having symptoms for several years after, Lyme is the number one vector-borne disease. While antibiotics are helpful and are said to resolve the issue, many people have continued symptoms even though the disease can't be conclusively identified. This persistent post-treatment Lyme disease syndrome responds well to the Protocol. It seems the storehouse for the infection remains in the gut, or perhaps the infection alters whatever form of chronic intestinal infection was already present. When intestinal infection is cleared with enzymes and the rest of the Protocol is followed, the full range of related symptoms improve. History of Lyme disease makes people especially sensitive to eating the common food irritants. To reduce symptoms, these patients often must be particularly careful about their diet and other aspects of the Protocol.

Migraines

All patients of the last few years who have carefully followed the Protocol have eliminated their migraines as long as they carefully avoid the four common food irritants. There are no established effective treatments for migraines, so my claim may sound unlikely. All patients with a history or present condition of migraines react negatively to corn, cow dairy, soy, and gluten. When the Protocol is followed, foods that previously triggered migraines, such as chocolate and caffeine, can usually be reintroduced. When explaining the role of the four food irritants, part of me wants to apologize, but part of me recognizes it may be the best and most important news a person has ever received. The results are relatively easy for a motivated person to confirm for themselves by following the Protocol.

Narcolepsy

I've only had one patient with severe narcolepsy, but the results were so profound that they should be mentioned. I've had multiple other patients who were either diagnosed with this condition or who would quickly fall asleep if they sat down in the early evening to watch media. They resolved as well. One patient was spending five hundred dollars per month on stimulants just to function and work. He managed the condition for many years. Less than two months into care, he was fine without medication. I didn't see him for about six years, but when he came back, he was still free of the condition. The treatment is to address the seven causes of disease.

Insomnia

It's difficult or perhaps impossible to maintain health without adequate sleep. Lack of sleep increases the risk of most health conditions. Taking pharmaceuticals or powerful herbs that may induce a sleep-like state always has side effects and isn't the same as sleep. Of course, lying awake at night can be very frustrating, and understandably, people look for a chemical solution. Unfortunately, chemicals, melatonin, and powerful herbs don't create health or healthy sleep.

The entire Protocol is relevant to sleep, but elevated cortisol, overconsumption of carbohydrates, and poor absorption of minerals are especially important components. Cortisol is driven by blood sugar instability and the related stress to the adrenals (Chapter 6) and from the stress that presents as weakness of the pancreas (Chapter 9). People rarely realize that skipping meals or having coffee on an empty stomach in the morning can cause sleeplessness at night. Not walking and/or eating too much carbohydrate and/or exercising too hard too frequently can prevent sleep as well. Walking reduces cortisol and appears to be the most effective way to clear sugar from the blood. If we are stewing in sugar, why would we be able to sleep? Elevated cortisol suppresses digestion, which interferes with our ability to absorb minerals and vitamin B12 needed to calm the nervous system and fall asleep. The other thing that might put you to sleep is listening to this as an audiobook.

The stimulating effect of even decaf coffee or chocolate affects people to varying degrees. Some people easily and quickly metabolize these components or are simply unaffected by them and can sleep after a big cup of coffee. The Protocol enables people to drink moderate amounts of caffeine without negative symptoms, but it also seems patients become more aware of sleep disturbance caused by ingesting stimulants less than four to six hours before bed. I used to be able to eat a truckload of chocolate just before bed, but now with a quarter of a dark chocolate bar after four p.m., sleep is compromised. This increased sensitivity to stimulants is probably because I'm no longer overloaded with sugar and cortisol—but attaining fifty contributes as well.

I find if I sleep more than eight hours, which I'm inclined to do, I may lie awake for some time the following night. Usually, I set an alarm to avoid oversleeping. I'd rather wake up early and be productive than lie awake the next night with a wandering mind or trying to quiet the mind with meditation. Meditating lying down, rather than being frustrated or concerned about the next day, is free of negative side effects, yields the benefits of meditation, and it can work almost as well as sleep as far as the next day is concerned.

Addiction and Depression

I lump these together because they're examples of conditions I don't claim to treat, but by addressing systemic issues, they usually become much easier to manage or no longer require additional management. Sometimes addiction and depression fall into the category of a "brain chemistry issue" that many manage with a prescription or self-medication, or these conditions may be driven by low energy, pain, and dysfunction. It's known that brain chemistry issues are driven by hormones, blood sugar swings, deficiencies, and the inability to clear chemicals from the system. Eventually, it will be known widely that corn sensitivity and its effect on the brain and pituitary are critical factors as well. Solving these issues at a causative level may address the inability to make enough of a particular neurotransmitter or heal various forms of brain trauma or emotional trauma. Helping a person to have more energy, decrease pain, and walk more sets the stage for this healing. Some studies show walking to be more effective than antidepressants.

Patients often tell me that their other doctors or practitioners insist that until they quit smoking or drinking or other addictions, they won't be able to address their symptoms. I find it can be the other way around. If people can feel better, have more energy, and walk, it may be easier to break an addiction. Cravings driven by blood sugar instability and eating too much sugar often seem to contribute to a variety of addictions.

A patient recently came to my office in tears of joy. Her long list of symptoms had cleared up in the first six weeks of care, or five office visits. The biggest symptoms resolved were her depression and anxiety, which weren't why she came to me and she never imagined we could improve. With one or two more visits over the next six weeks, we were done with active care because she knows how to eat, how to exercise, and what simple, mostly food-based supplements to take to keep her symptoms from coming back. Occasional checkups help to ensure it stays that way.

Anxiety/Panic/Heartbeat Irregularities

I lump these together because it seems their primary driver is mineral/electrolyte deficiency or imbalance. I don't claim to treat anxiety or panic attacks. Certainly, these issues can be driven in part by personality, history, or situation. That said, every time I work with people with panic attacks, one month into care the attacks are either gone or at least 80 percent reduced in frequency and/or severity. Heartbeat irregularities are perhaps more variable, but when people follow the Protocol, this issue becomes less severe or resolves. Addressing absorption issues and using food-source minerals consistently resolves deficiencies and related symptoms.

I worked with a successful professional who was in the process of planning a move from the San Francisco Bay Area because he thought the abundance of electromagnetic fields (EMFs) was the cause of his anxiety. To control his symptoms, he was on a moderate to high dose of a powerful med, which created unpleasant side effects. One month into care he said his anxiety was gone and he was off his medication. He suddenly faced a new problem: he didn't know what to do; his anxiety had been organizing and motivating his life for a long time. Two weeks later he reported he was doing well and was now adapting to a life without anxiety. His symptoms didn't return in the few years in which we followed up occasionally. While I have some skepticism about EMFs causing symptoms, we know that many people are highly sensitive to components that have no effects on others. Did he have anxiety because of mineral deficiency or imbalance, or did that imbalance make him extra sensitive to EMFs? Not an easy question to answer conclusively, but anxiety usually significantly improves or resolves with the Protocol.

Chapter 14

Solving Kids' Issues

Eczema, Poor Appetite, Nightmares, Frequent Illness, Etcetera

The Protocol is gentle enough to be used with babies and children, and the results tend to come even quicker and easier than with adults. It's helpful when parents are also on the Protocol or at least the same diet. If parents realize they themselves don't benefit from excess carbs in their diet and that they may even be addicted to them, they are more likely to be able to guide their kids in a better diet. Sometimes parents are concerned that they are depriving their kids when they reduce their carbs. Often, this dietary change creates significant improvements in health, mental clarity, behavior, and reduction of colds and flu—greater gifts than sweets and grains. Sometimes carbs aren't the most important issue for a particular kid's health, especially if they are very active and eat a reasonable diet, so parents may not have to go there.

Most kids with health issues have intestinal infection. They may pick it up at birth, in the hospital, or from the wrong handful of dirt. Because almost everyone is deficient in zinc, the same is true of newborns. This means they also have weak stomach acid and are vulnerable to intestinal infection.

These problems, combined with eating foods we weren't designed to eat, explains most of the common issues of this age group. Whether newborns are nursing from mothers who eat the common food irritants or drink formula made from these subsidized foods, most babies are exposed to problematic foods or their mothers' reactions to these foods starting in utero.

By strengthening stomach acid, clearing intestinal infection, and switching to a better diet, we significantly improve or resolve colic, spitting up, eczema, rashes, poor appetite, bellyaches, and frequent illness. Adding minerals that can be absorbed resolves issues such as nightmares, growing pains, and leg cramps. This step at least helps anxiety and bedwetting, but these issues can be driven more by personality and situation.

Kids with poor appetites or very picky eaters are quite satisfying to treat. With the basic foundation of this approach in place, I've always seen these issues improve dramatically. I worked with a five-year-old who only ate cheese and pasta. She wouldn't even eat blueberries. Two weeks into the Protocol she started to eat raw turnips, chicken, broccoli, and even blueberries. Chronic intestinal infection and weak stomach acid may cause swings in appetite or other eating issues. These people may be very hungry, but after two bites of food, they can no longer eat, or they may be extra sensitive to the smells or tastes of certain foods.

Kids or adults who often get sick benefit greatly from this protocol. From as early as I can remember until I started to put these pieces together in my late thirties, I used to get multiple colds every year, and I would spend at least a week on the couch with the flu. My wife was in a similar state. Now we rarely get sick. If we do it's mild. Our daughters win gift certificates (for ice cream) at their grade school for near-perfect attendance. This illustrates that frequent illness ran in our families because of diet and intestinal infection, not because of a genetically determined issue.

Genetics are blamed for many conditions that are actually environmental—diet and intestinal infection are the main environmental components rarely identified or addressed. We demonstrate this point when we clear the same health issue suffered by multiple generations of a family. They probably all had the same form of intestinal infection and similar diets. They thought their digestive issues, migraines, arthritis, allergies, dysmenorrhea, etcetera were genetically determined, and maybe it was genetically determined that they were more likely to develop sensitivities to food irritants or that intestinal infection would affect them in a particular way.

Because acne tends to be an issue for teenagers, it may be more difficult implementing the diet to clear the skin. Compliance and the ability to follow the Protocol can be challenging at this age. If kids choose to eat "normal food" at school or elsewhere, it may be difficult to achieve a full resolution. When compliance is good and people are patient and able to follow up a few times over a couple of months, good results with most skin conditions can be expected. If we can at least strengthen stomach acid, clear intestinal infection, and possibly improve the diet at home, their health will improve over time, perhaps resolving symptoms or at least helping them to see that a solution is available.

Dysmenorrhea (also see Chapter 12), or difficult menstrual cycles, is a common complaint of girls and women. People rarely get a solution to this issue that doesn't involve the addition of potentially dangerous pharmaceuticals. Often, the issue is written off as being "normal" or "it runs in the family," but we consistently resolve this issue. Having periods free of negative symptoms without adding synthetic hormones or painkillers to the body leads to better overall health and the possible prevention of a wide variety of hormone-related issues, such as osteoporosis, infertility, problems with pregnancy, and a variety of cancers. The possibility of avoiding these issues may be inspiring, but the immediate results of easing the monthly cycle may be life-changing in and of itself.

Another poorly treated issue that usually has its onset around this age is scoliosis. While I don't know if I could help a patient successfully prevent or treat scoliosis, I don't see anyone else offering great solutions. My model, based on the foundation of applied kinesiology, could explain the muscle weakness and instability that leads to severe lateral curvature of the spine. While the use of back braces and spinal surgery are the main current options, they can be dangerous, ineffective, or lead to a variety of other problems. If we could address muscle weakness caused by internal issues early in the progression of this deformity, we might be able to stabilize the spine and prevent advancement to scoliosis. This would require identifying the issue early and monitoring for further progression.

CHAPTER 15
Athletic Performance

One of the most important factors in becoming a great athlete is avoiding injury and illness so that consistent training and event participation can be maintained. The recent alarming increase in injuries for even non-contact sports points to a universal problem. Increased general inflammation is leading to debilitating injuries, repetitive stress injuries, and concussions, all of which now affect more, and younger, people. Surgical remedies such as the Tommy John or ulnar collateral ligament reconstruction (elbow repair) are rapidly becoming more common. High school sports injuries derail the athletic futures of too many young people. Every time an athlete gets injured or sick, training stalls or regresses, or their career may be over.

By identifying and clearing numerous muscle weaknesses, people become stronger, faster, and more coordinated. This is great for putting groceries in the car, playing competitive sports, or backcountry skiing. Athletes who carefully measure their performance (weightlifting, timed events, etc.) are rewarding to work with because the results are measurable. Working with adolescents or younger athletes is fantastic because the rate at which they improve is stunning, and the difference it makes in their lives is inspiring.

One very inspiring athlete I've worked with is Evan Strong. He's a snowboarder who lost a leg in a motorcycle accident when he was eighteen. At the Sochi 2014 Winter Paralympics, Evan was the only U.S. individual gold medalist. The day before the race in Sochi, the Russian hosts invited Evan and his teammates to a complimentary meal at one of the most famous American fast food restaurants conveniently located nearby. Through our work together, Evan had seen the impact of even small amounts of the common food irritants, and he declined to eat any of the not-so-happy meal. His teammates felt poorly after the free lunch, and the next day, Evan was on the top of the podium by a very narrow margin.

With this protocol people heal, performance improves, and athletes show up consistently for their sports. Atmospheric CO_2 is increasing, food quality is decreasing, and people walk less. These conditions create inflammation, poor absorption, and hormone imbalance that exacerbate joint injuries and concussions, calcium deficiency that drives shin splints and plantar fasciitis, elevated cortisol that contributes to poor healing, repetitive stress injuries, colds and flu, and muscle weaknesses that make people vulnerable to injury and slow or impossible to heal.

I work with a college softball pitcher who was limited by low back pain. She was okay as long as she didn't pitch. She'd gone to multiple doctors and practitioners with minimal results. Six weeks into the Protocol, her pain was gone, and she was back to star-pitcher status. But she got tired of eating carefully, and so her pain returned. She came back to see me, and we cleared it again, but then she went back to a poor diet, and she came back again. She didn't want to believe she had to follow my guidelines to pitch like a monster, but she proved it to herself, repeatedly. It's worth it because she loves pitching. She sees her teammates struggle with injuries and illness, but without this book, it's hard for them to understand how this could be possible. Diet alone wouldn't have been a solution because chronic intestinal infection weakened her psoas muscles causing a significant portion of her low back tension. Elevated cortisol created inflammation. Overtraining and not walking stressed the pancreas, weakening the latissimi dorsi and further compromising back strength.

To ensure the Protocol has the greatest impact on overall health, it's best implemented in full. Selecting pieces that "fit" into a person's lifestyle may or may not achieve results.

Chapter 16

Obstacles: It's Hard to Be Human

During moments of uncertainty I tend to focus on missed opportunities and patients who were unable to hang in there and achieve a positive result. It's disappointing when people disappear six weeks into care and won't return a phone call. I dwell on it at times. Of course, everyone has their own lives to live, and we can only do what we can do and only when we're ready to do it, but I'm a fan of communication and follow-through—even when it's difficult. Conversely, I sometimes forget to reflect on the lives of all the people I've helped over the years. How many of them have improved the quality of their life and have resolved or avoided a variety of serious health conditions? How has this changed the course of their lives and of all their relations? When I run into a patient I haven't seen for a few years, who once suffered from migraines half the time and now has none, I have the opportunity to consider my impact on their lives. With this book, I am creating the possibility of countless others resolving symptoms and a path for my patients to understand and succeed with the Protocol for Health.

Depending on your perspective, the Protocol may not be easy.

Unsustainability is a common complaint by dieticians, even for diets that are less challenging than mine. When patients resolve serious conditions using the Protocol and see that their symptoms are determined by their diet, this way of life suddenly seems essential and sustainable. However, especially at the beginning of care, people may not be able to sustain this diet. They may develop unhealthy feelings about themselves or about food unless they make choices to avoid being overwhelmed. The Protocol isn't made up of ideas or rules I created; it became apparent through the observation of patterns of muscle weakness associated with internal issues that resolve when the seven causes of disease are addressed. It's about making choices and determining what effort is worthwhile for an individual. If a patient can't eat ham and eggs or a similar protein-rich breakfast because of nausea or repulsion, they may need to eat something else and retry that meal later. A low-carb rice protein drink with coconut milk, corn-free vanilla, and stevia might be easier for them. Maybe it won't yield as much benefit as quickly as an ideal breakfast, but it's better than having a terrible breakfast experience or giving up on this system altogether.

Sometimes patients want my "permission" to break some "rule," but these aren't rules; they are guidelines that have proven to be effective. People can choose whether they want to follow them. When all of the conditions are met, people consistently break out of an extraordinary variety of health conditions. Sometimes the results are achieved without all the pieces being in place, and sometimes people have to be patient with themselves and their results until they're ready to follow all the guidelines.

Looking at all of the pieces of this system at the same time can be overwhelming. Some long-term patients admit that, while it's clearly worthwhile and sustainable now, had they known about the full picture at the beginning, they might not have started.

They, along with me, had the opportunity to ease into this system because we didn't know all the pieces back then. If we were lucky, the first couple of pieces worked well enough to confirm that we had at least found a partial solution. But without all the pieces, it's uncertain whether the results will be achieved. New patients don't have to do it all at once. They can choose the parts they're ready for. If they continue to add more pieces of the Protocol over time, they can improve their chances of achieving a better result sooner. If a piece isn't adequately applied, it is made apparent through testing and shows us where to focus our efforts if we're motivated to improve further.

My process of creating and following the Protocol is one of patience, trial and error, incremental progress, and mistakes as well as gratitude for the fact that I don't suffer from the health issues of my past. Its significance for my family is impossible to fully realize. If we didn't have the health to care for ourselves, each other, our family, home, land, animals, and office—how would it work? Too many people have to answer these questions. It's challenging to guide people toward better health without being overly attached to the outcome when it's clear how powerful this solution is and how much is at stake.

If I show a kid how to clear her eczema, will she realize that the same changes could greatly simplify her future health and help her become a star athlete or avoid acne or colds and flu or more significant issues in life? I think so. I hope so.

One of the greatest challenges in my practice is to help people see the big picture of this process. Even if someone resolves significant pain, will they understand and remember that I can help them with their digestion or some other issue in the future? If their pain returns, will they think the Protocol didn't work, or will they come back so we can determine what component has drifted out of balance?

Understanding, remembering, and applying the components of the Protocol can be challenging enough; but when patients face deeper issues regarding cravings, addictions, traditions, cultures, religions, strong ideologies, or personal myths about health, the Protocol can be confusing or impossible.

Mostly, this method requires the will to try something different and be persistent. Not everyone can do that or may need to do that; but for those who are motivated to try this system, managing the obstacles is a personal process that may require additional assistance. Fortunately, this process helps people become stronger, have more energy, and have greater mental clarity. These benefits enable people to see the value of the Protocol for Health and realize that they can achieve and sustain what previously seemed unlikely or impossible.

When it's understood that carbohydrates drive most addictions and that the craving for carbohydrates is caused by blood sugar instability, a lack of mild aerobic exercise, and chronic intestinal infection, the interconnected and holistic nature of this system becomes clear. But are those pieces more important than the effects of poor absorption of nutrients, inflammation, and the effects of corn on the brain and the pituitary gland? It depends on the individual, but the parts of the Protocol all work together.

The interconnectedness of the components of this system enable rapid healing, possibly without a pop, or a dramatic treatment, but occur naturally from the inside with the removal of obstacles to health. This is half the reason I take detailed notes in practice. When people eliminate symptoms, they often forget they ever had them. I might ask about their knee pain, and they have to pause and think as they realize they were unaware of its disappearance. Unfortunately, this means people frequently explain away the resolution of their symptoms and give credit to an exercise posture, tropical berries, good posture, or anything other than the Protocol clearing obstacles to their healing. While people may benefit from some other complementary component, especially once we have started to clear weaknesses and other issues, the Protocol consistently stands on its own for the resolution of symptoms. To not realize that is a missed opportunity.

Even within this system, people often give credit to just one component. Because we strengthen stomach acid and clear intestinal infection at the beginning of care, patients don't realize the diet alone might not have helped, or at least not as much, without those pieces in place. Without strengthening stomach acid, they might have no appetite for a simple diet. Without walking, they'll remain extra sensitive to carbohydrates and food irritants. Without supplements to address vitamin and mineral deficiencies, they will have associated muscle weaknesses and they won't feel as well, and without zinc and HCl, absorption of nutrients will be minimal and intestinal infection will return. The adrenal diet affects everything. How can you consistently heal or balance hormones without stabilizing blood sugar and reducing cortisol? Until muscle injuries are cleared, an error in the diet may exacerbate an old injury. Any of the seven causes of disease can create symptoms, but none of their solutions, on their own, are likely to create a lasting resolution of symptoms. People don't realize how simple and effective healthcare can be, but most of the Protocol depends on the rest of the Protocol, which can make it simple but complicated.

Friends and family of my patients mostly just see how carefully food choices are made, but until one proves it to oneself, the diet may seem difficult and unlikely to be so important. For people with mild or no symptoms, the Protocol may not create noticeable changes and may not seem worth the effort, unless a person is especially motivated to avoid the normal premature decline of health. Many people, even those with serious digestive issues, may still be unwilling to try a simple diet, but since no known treatment works consistently, can you blame them? If it seems like a stretch that diet and a related protocol could be effective with digestive issues, then the idea that corn can cause mental illness and tennis elbow may be slow to gain traction. Even if corn only causes mental fog for an individual, that fog is an obstacle to this protocol. Since corn is the number one subsidized food and therefore the number one food additive, we have a problem.

Another obstacle to this regimen is the desire we all have to be entertained. When food and exercise are entertainment, people don't want a simple solution. In the past, we walked as a means of transportation, so walking wouldn't have been part of the Protocol, but now we have to go out of our way to create sustained mild aerobic exercise. Whether it's always doing the same walk or walking on a treadmill, exercise boredom is an issue for most of us. For me to stay on a treadmill for forty minutes, I need some additional entertainment. Exercise classes are designed to be entertaining, but exercise classes are filled with components that could never be maintained for forty minutes, so they're not a substitute for sustained mild aerobic exercise. Sometimes I get bored with simple meat, eggs, vegetables, goat cheese, coconut products, butter, and the few other things I eat. I like to eat more entertaining food, and though millions of recipes fit my guidelines, I usually don't want to prepare them. So, I eat simply and repetitively or poison myself with mainstream food or mostly find some happy middle ground that involves family, friends, and/or the rare-risky-expensive prepared food that may fit the Protocol for Health.

For many people, entertainment also includes diets, healthcare, and new fancy supplements. If they find a system that actually works, but it focuses on simple components (boring) and self-discipline (more boring), will they be able to stay with it? Of course, it's smart to keep looking for ways to fine-tune and improve our health, but too often my patients create negative symptoms as they try new diets, supplements, "superfoods," "adaptogens," and protein drinks. Ideally, we talk before they try these, or in the case of an unusual supplement or food, we test patients directly to these items. Most supplements test poorly, and most long lists of ingredients contain some sort of detectable irritant. Keeping it simple and within guidelines identified through an individual's nervous system can avoid setbacks and wasted time, effort, and expense.

When it's important to a patient to try something new, it can be quite valuable to get feedback through their own nervous system. For instance, if a patient decides they want to become vegetarian, the biggest obstacle is how to get enough protein without eating too many carbohydrates. By balancing how much they walk (or similar exercise) with how much they turn to nuts and goat cheese for protein, we may be able to keep them healthy on a vegetarian diet. If they eat too many carbs or don't walk enough, the pancreas will be stressed, and their lats will be weak. If they don't eat enough protein, the stress to the adrenals will weaken three muscles that cross the knee. If they start to react to nuts from eating them too frequently or because of added chemicals, we can confirm it with in-office testing. The same evaluation can be applied to intermittent fasting, intense physical training, or whether frequent hot yoga or drinking a pot of coffee per day works for an individual. In a world where there is no consensus on vegetarian versus carnivore, fats versus carbohydrates, cardio or high-intensity, ideal protein quantities, or foods to avoid, these definitive answers are extraordinary.

Are you open to the possibility that there is a way to obtain information directly from the body that guides a path to transform your health and medical future? Most of us have our expectations of an ordinary health outcome: premature health decline with *ordinary* aches and pains and a wide variety of *ordinary* diseases to choose from. So, when your doctor, or whoever, says you'll just have to learn to live with the pain or risk your life with drugs and surgery, it's true—for ordinary. How ordinary do we want to be?

    I have faith in the human body, and I see untapped potential in our nervous systems. Many smart people have worked in healthcare for a long time, and while specialization has illuminated so much, it also creates blind spots and incongruity. Clear answers through our nervous system guide a clear path to health. In some ways, it is strange that the Protocol for Health is made of such simple pieces; but then again, why wouldn't a real solution be simple?

Acknowledgments

My wife and daughters are the center of my life. They are also tremendous support in nurturing our health, home, and livelihood. Without the foundation of their support, it is unlikely this project could ever have been completed.

My parents continue to actively support my family and work. The privilege they have afforded has given me space and time to grow and develop all aspects of my life, the Protocol, my practice, and this book.

Being in practice for sixteen years with my mother, Dr. Jeanne Archer, has been remarkably positive and enriching. Early on, when I was unwilling to proceed with a patient's care without certainty, she helped me to establish clarity. Together we have developed and honed our practices to better serve the health needs of our patients. She has been invaluable in validating my system of muscle testing and the resultant solutions our practice has incorporated. The more clearly this system defines the seven underlying causes of disease, the more our work is about encouraging people to change their lives and patterns. She has led by example by confronting obstacles and injustice for the health of anyone in need.

I'm grateful for all of my teachers and all teachers who share knowledge, wisdom, and insight as well as those of past generations: teachers, doctors, and medicine people. It is a gift to have their encouragement, or simply tolerance, as they show, or we ask, *how they know*—so that we have something valuable to share with our patients and all of our relations. Dr. George Goodhart and the founders/developers of applied kinesiology have blended ancient mystery with modern science to create a new understanding of the body. The teachers of the International College of Applied Kinesiology further organize, contribute, and share. Dr. Phil Maffetone built on that foundation with detailed work with athletes, diet, and heart rate monitors to create a book that helped to transform my health, guide part of my protocol, and restore the health and innate athletic ability of many. That book has evolved into *The Big Book of Health and Fitness*. Author scholars Dr. Loren Cordain, Robb Wolf, Mark Sisson, and others have come to some of the same conclusions as they approach issues from the perspective of Ancestral Health informed by biochemistry. Their development and support of Paleo and ketogenic diets have launched a movement that is being validated by a rising tide of grateful, inspired followers and clinical research. Acupuncturist Stephen Barr and his Conscious Healing courses offer a bridge from the mystical to the objective that has simplified and strengthened my protocol.

I'm constantly inspired by the willingness of my patients to try. People with common or terrible issues who have tried many doctors and modalities and are still willing to try again, and to share their feelings and mystery within. These conversations with new patients and those who are in their second decade of care change me and lift me from common concerns. People established in care inspire me to share and expect miracles with new patients; observing consistent miracles shows me they are not miracles but predictable results of a complete Protocol for Health, which I know only because of the willingness of patients to try. They give me the gift of confidence and knowing I have something worth sharing.

Patients like Rene, Tina, Dianne, and Anthony have had a tremendous impact on my life and practice. These people have developed their own communities of support as they inspire others with their understanding, generosity, and integrity. They keep me connected to many patients, helping me to see the long-term benefits for those they inspire. SuAnn, who has helped to run our office for many years, has brought continual positivity, new ideas, and warmth to our practice. She holds a space for us and our patients that enables our work on many levels.

Bringing in the right editors at the right time dramatically improved my productivity and helped me to move forward with inspiration. Dimitri Keriotis walked a great balance of corrections, observation, and encouragement. Cynthia Schmidt has been incredibly generous with her time and expertise and has brought further clarity to this project. My family and friends have also contributed excellent feedback and suggestions: my wife Meghan and her parents, brother, and sister, my dad and Tom, and Leeza and Nico.

Appendix A

A Study of Cow Dairy and Low Back Pain

A few years ago, I ran a study with a group of volunteers to demonstrate the connection between cow's milk dairy consumption and chronic low back pain. I chose to conduct this study because my technique revealed that dairy consumption weakens the psoas major muscles, which causes opposing tension in the low back, making people more likely to have low back pain and poor healing of low back injuries. I hoped that I could publish this study and help many people reduce their low back pain while I advanced my practice. While the twenty-eight people in the study significantly reduced their low back pain, I'm not a trained researcher, and I was unable to publish the study. Still, the benefits that most of those people received and what I learned in the process helped me to help others and made the process worthwhile.

My biggest realization since then is that chronic intestinal infection is an even greater cause of low back pain. However, the impact of dairy remains significant, and for a study, it's simpler to remove dairy from the diet than to clear intestinal infection. In general, if I meet people who have long-term low back pain, I encourage them to come to see me at the office because it's almost certain we can eliminate their pain. But sometimes I meet someone who can't or won't come to see me, so I just suggest they eliminate dairy products for at least a couple of months. Several of these people later told me they confirmed their low back pain was connected to or caused by dairy consumption, and their pain had decreased or resolved.

It would be great to repeat this study with the help of trained researchers to help some of the millions of people who suffer from low back pain. In the meantime, here's that study from a few years ago.

Low back pain linked to dairy product consumption: a case series.

J. Matthew Archer, D.C.
Archer Chiropractic, Nevada City, California, U.S.
An Independent Study

Background

This study involves only the elimination of dairy products from the diets of people with chronic low back pain. This single food elimination diet is based on the finding that, under specific conditions, almost all patients with recurring or chronic low back pain present with neurologically inhibited (weak) psoas muscles. This weakness of the deep hip flexors or "core strength" muscles can be demonstrated through manual muscle testing. Specific chiropractic adjustments can temporarily strengthen the psoai, but the elimination of dairy products from the diet causes lasting facilitation of the psoas muscles and a decrease or elimination of low back pain. This testing is possible because of a breakthrough in the technique of Applied Kinesiology (AK).

Methods

To test this hypothesis, twenty-eight people with chronic low back pain (ongoing low back pain for at least six months) removed dairy products from their diets for eight weeks, and their scores on the Oswestry Disability Index (ODI) questionnaires [1] were compared from the start to the end of eight weeks. There was no clinical examination, treatment, or muscle testing of the participants before or during the study. Volunteers were solicited by newspaper announcements. There was no control or randomization.

Results

Overall the participants (n=28) averaged a 34 percent improvement in low back pain. Four people had 100 percent improvement from scores of 8, 18, 22, and 32 percent disability. Over half of the subjects averaged a 70 percent improvement in their ODI scores during the eight-week study. Twenty-one of the subjects improved their low back pain, while one person was unchanged, and six subjects finished the study with more pain than when they started.

Conclusions

While this study is a simple case series with limited implications, it supports what is seen in practice: many people with chronic low back pain improve significantly when they eliminate cow dairy products from the diet.

Keywords

Low back pain; chronic low back pain; dairy products; single food elimination diet; Applied Kinesiology; food allergy; food sensitivity; psoas muscle inhibition; manual muscle testing; chiropractic adjustment; Oswestry Disability Index.

Background

While it remains scientifically unclear if manual muscle testing as applied by the chiropractic technique of AK is valid [2,3], the results of this study support the validity of the technique.

AK considers any joint pain or dysfunction in terms of muscle balance. If a muscle on one side of a joint is neurologically inhibited (weak), then the antagonistic muscle(s) may become spastic and painful. This reciprocal contraction is explained as a means of stabilizing an unbalanced joint [4]. Applying this model to the low back, pain in the area of the extensor muscles is likely to be caused by inhibition of hip and trunk flexor muscles. If the psoas muscles are inhibited, there is often pain or tension in or near the quadratus lumborum muscles of the lumbar spine. Some people find that if they do sit-ups, crunches, or other core-strengthening exercises regularly, it helps to control their low back pain. From the perspective of the AK model, they are strengthening the abdominals to compensate for inhibited psoas muscles. If the psoai are inhibited, repeated forward bends (like gardening) stretch already-tight low back muscles that may cause low back pain. If dairy products are causing inhibition of the psoai in dairy-sensitive individuals, low back pain often decreases when milk products are removed from the diet. The association between a reduced disability outcome of chronic low back pain and reduced dairy intake can be confirmed through this testing method, supported by clinical findings, and can be demonstrated by testing study subjects before and after dairy elimination (which was not a component of this study).

The breakthrough that led to this study involves establishing a clear baseline from which to begin manual muscle testing. This approach makes it possible to observe a clear distinction between neurologically facilitated or inhibited (strong or weak) muscles or to pre and post strength test any semi-isolated muscle. This baseline for testing is established in about five minutes by identifying and addressing eight different factors that interfere with muscle testing. It is then possible to demonstrate muscle weakness when a dairy-sensitive person has a small sample of dairy product placed in their mouth. A demonstration can be made using a small, untrained (in AK) adult to test a large athlete with a history of recurring or chronic low back pain or known lactose intolerance. Once a trained practitioner has addressed these eight factors, a strength test to dairy products is possible. Some false negative tests are possible initially, but after a few office visits and the application of certain therapies, these can be resolved.

It is important to note that there is controversy surrounding AK and manual muscle testing. One can go online and find arguments and demonstrations for and against AK, and unfortunately both proponents and opponents often demonstrate techniques that are not recognized by the International College of Applied Kinesiology. Also, practitioners with good intentions can be misled with inaccurate muscle testing. In the hands of a capable doctor, excellent results are possible. Training and certification are offered by the ICAK.

A review of research finds no previous studies linking dairy products with low back pain. Almost all adults in the U.S. experience low back pain at some time and the cause of that pain can rarely be determined [6]. When low back pain becomes chronic, it usually persists for years [7]. This case series is presented to initiate a breakthrough in our understanding of low back pain and the role of food reactions in the bigger picture of healthcare.

Methods

To find participants with chronic low back pain for this study, announcements were placed in the local newspaper. The notice stated that the study would involve removing one common food from the diet for eight weeks and would not involve any physical contact. Subjects consented into the study in groups of two to eight, and the study procedure was described in detail including why it was expected to relieve low back pain. Subjects were told to eliminate cow dairy products (any food made from cow's milk) from the diet for eight weeks. Intake included the first ODI. Subjects were sent home with instructions to complete four more ODIs after one, two, four, and eight weeks. Take-home packets also included a description of dairy products to be eliminated. Subjects were called four times during the study to discuss their progress and to ask if they were able to keep dairy products out of their diet. If they claimed the consumption of some dairy product, participants were again encouraged to eliminate it. Participants' self-reported compliance was high, and none claimed to consume dairy more than six times during the eight weeks. One participant was excluded from the study because they had been unknowingly eating dairy products daily and then was unwilling to eliminate that food. Sixteen subjects dropped out of the study, all but one within one week of starting. Twenty-eight participants completed the eight-week study.

Because most butter does not trigger psoas muscle inhibition [5], the study participants were free to consume it during the eight-week study. Butter is mostly milk fat that seems free of (or very low in) the provocative proteins. Goat and sheep dairy products were to be excluded for the duration of the study. In clinical practice I observe that these alternatives to cow's milk cause weakening of the psoai in less than 10 percent of patients who react to cow's milk. Raw dairy products, and dairy products with lactose removed, both cause psoas weakness and were excluded from the diet for this study.

The changes in ODI scores were measured between the day-one introduction and the end of eight weeks. The test scores at one, two, and four weeks were used to monitor the participants' low back pain and did not enter into calculations. The tests were scored according to the standard directions for the ODI. In the rare event that two boxes were checked for a single question and the respondents' intention was not indicated, the box of greater disability was counted.

Although the design of this study is based on observations from clinical practice that incorporates manual muscle testing, there was no manual muscle testing involved in the study. I include findings and discussion of manual muscle testing to show why I chose to design the study as is and to illustrate the use of this technique in practice. Describing the eight factors I check to establish a baseline from which to begin manual muscle testing and how this differs from that taught by the ICAK is beyond the scope of this paper.

Presentation of case series participants

All adult study subjects were included in this study, as long as they had low back pain for at least six months, and they ate dairy products at least four times per week on average. The average age of the study participants was fifty-nine, and their histories included back surgery, disc injuries, spinal fractures, diabetes, heart disease, emphysema, cancer, obesity, hepatitis, etcetera. Perhaps a younger group of participants with less complicated conditions would show a greater average improvement in low back pain with the same single food elimination diet.

Results

Overall the participants (n=28) averaged a 34 percent improvement in low back pain. Four people had 100 percent improvement from scores of 8, 18, 22, and 32 percent disability. Over half of the subjects averaged a 70 percent improvement in their ODI scores during the eight-week study. Twenty-one of the subjects improved their low back pain, while one person was unchanged, and six subjects finished the study with more pain than when they started.

A frequency plot of percentage improvement per participant (see graph) yields a bimodal distribution curve of subject outcome. This curve shows that eleven out of twenty-eight subjects had an improvement in low back pain of 67 percent or greater which fell outside of a normal bell curve.

Graph

Frequency plot—how frequently did a participant improve by a certain percentage.

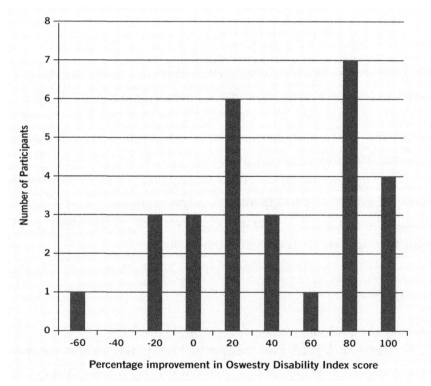

Discussion

The data show that over half of the subjects averaged a 70 percent improvement in low back pain during the study. When graphed as a frequency plot, it is apparent that for a certain group of people with chronic low back pain, excluding dairy products from the diet could significantly improve symptoms. Because there was no control group, uncertainty remains as to whether the elimination of dairy products would have this impact on the general population with chronic low back pain. Still, many of the participants and others who have removed dairy products from their diets report improved low back pain that returns when they ingest dairy products.

This study offers a possible solution to low back pain that can be applied with no financial cost and no known health risk. While this study may be insufficient for establishing this single food elimination diet as a therapy for low back pain, why not just try it? While it may be inconvenient to eliminate dairy products from the diet, an individual can determine if it makes a difference in their pain. Although some may be concerned about a lack of calcium without dairy products, this concern can be addressed with other foods or calcium supplements and should not prevent an eight-week dietary test. According to The Harvard School of Public Health, there are risks associated with high dairy consumption and questions about the effectiveness of dairy products for preventing osteoporosis [8]. For those who suffer frequent, constant, or debilitating low back pain, the potential benefits of eliminating dairy products from the diet certainly outweigh any inconvenience or short-term dietary losses.

While just over half the participants had a significant improvement during the study, I observe in practice that about 95 percent of people with recurring or chronic low back pain react to dairy products. Other complicating factors in addition to dairy reaction likely prevented some of the subjects from experiencing improvement during the study. However, some subjects whose low back pain didn't improve during the study noticed other benefits, such as decreases in seasonal allergies, heartburn, and/or headaches. These side benefits suggest that even though a subject's low back pain did not improve, they may indeed react to dairy products. This form of testing can also link low back pain to blood sugar issues, intestinal conditions, mineral deficiencies, and muscle injuries. Addressing these issues, combined with the elimination of dairy products and supported with known effective therapies, I observe that patients receive lasting relief from chronic low back pain.

I hypothesize that this method of testing dairy products (and other foods) yields insights into genetically linked reactions to proteins related to food sensitivity and/or food allergy. However, because there are no known accurate tests for reactions to foods, this is difficult to confirm. A review of available testing methods (IgE, IgG, pinprick, scratch, and genetic testing) all show false positives and false negatives and frequently lack correlation with an individual's symptoms [9-12]. The lack of accurate testing is illustrated by what is considered the "gold standard" of food allergy testing: food challenge. This test involves medical supervision while a patient consumes the suspected food allergen to observe the patient's symptoms. This method is the best medical test available but, considering that people with known food allergies sometimes consume an allergen without experiencing symptoms, it appears to have limited accuracy. While one study showed insight into the determination of food allergies using AK [13], it seems there has been more effort expended in attempting to "disprove" this form of testing than to prove it. Indeed, several "studies" of AK were performed by people untrained in AK. Rather than try to prove or disprove AK, this case series offers an observation made in clinical practice using this form of manual muscle testing. This testing appears to detect food allergy, food sensitivity, and/or possibly a genetic component underlying these conditions. In any case, dietary changes guided by these observations yield excellent results, especially with conditions known to be associated with allergies, such as asthma, eczema, digestive issues, seasonal allergies, and hypersensitivities.

This study does not show how much improvement in low back pain was due to factors other than the elimination of dairy from the diet because there was no control group. This was minimized by including only subjects who had had ongoing low back pain for at least six months and who were not starting any other treatments. The study could be strengthened by repeating it with randomization and control, and while it would be ideal to have double-blind testing for a single food elimination study, it is highly impractical. Because this study depends on honest and careful self-regulation of the diet, it was necessary to motivate study participants by informing them as to the reasoning for the study. Thus, a bias and placebo effect must be considered. These effects are canceled to some degree because consciously or not, some participants were certainly eating some dairy products during the study. While the study has these limitations, the improvement in ODI scores shows reaction to dairy products to be an important consideration for chronic low back pain.

Conclusions

This study shows a link between low back pain and the consumption of dairy products. A breakthrough in manual muscle testing and techniques borrowed from AK led to this discovery. Effective use of AK could transform how we look at the diet and the underlying causes of disease. If reactions to common foods could be linked to previously unconnected conditions (migraines, ADD/ADHD, digestive issues, arthritis, autoimmune conditions, etc.) healthcare could become more effective, simple, and safe.

While it may seem unlikely that dairy products could be linked to low back pain using current medically established testing methods, many people have experienced the connection for themselves. This study suggests that an individual has about a 50 percent chance of improving chronic low back pain in eight weeks or less by removing dairy products from their diet. Certainly, further study is needed, but a no-risk, no-cost treatment with a high rate of success may be the biggest breakthrough in low back pain to date.

Consent

Written informed consent was obtained from the participants for publication of this case series.

List of Abbreviations

AK – Applied Kinesiology
ICAK – International College of Applied Kinesiology
ODI – Oswestry Disability Index

Acknowledgments

It is an honor to acknowledge Dr. George Goodheart, D.C. as the founder of AK and for sharing his observation of the link between kidney dysfunction and psoas muscle inhibition.

I also wish to thank Dr. Dale Johnson, Ph.D., Director of Research at Life Chiropractic College West, and Dr. Malik Slosberg, D.C., M.S. for their generous advice and support.

REFERENCES

1. Fairbank JC, Pynsent PB: **The Oswestry Disability Index.** *Spine* 2000, **25**(22):2940-2953.

2. Cuthbert SC, Goodheart GJ: **On the reliability and validity of manual muscle testing: a literature review.** *Chiropr Man Therap* 2007, 15:4.

3. Haas M, Cooperstein R, and Peterson D: **Disentangling manual muscle testing and Applied Kinesiology: critique and reinterpretation of literature review.** Chiropr Man *Therap* 2007, 15:11.

4. Walther DS: **Applied Kinesiology, Synopsis. 2nd edition.** Pueblo, CO: Systems DC; 2000.

5. Francis T: *Applied Kinesiology Certification Course (Basic 100 Hour).* Santa Clara, CA. October 2000–May 2001.

6. National Institutes of Health, National Institute of Neurological Disorders and Stroke. Low Back Pain Fact Sheet. http://www.ninds.nih.gov/disorders/backpain/detail_backpain.htm#191273102

7. Hestbaek L, Leboeuf-Yde C, Engberg M, Lauritzen T, Bruun NH, Manniche C: **The course of low back pain in a general population. Results from a 5-year prospective study.** *J Manipulative Physiol Ther* 2003, **26**(4):213-9.

8. Harvard School of Public Health. http://www.hsph.harvard.edu/nutritionsource/what-should-you-eat/calcium-full-story/index.html

9. Fenton MJ, Sampson HA: Medscape Allergy and Immunology: What the New Food Allergy Guidelines Offer to Clinicians. http://www.medscape com/viewarticle/739532.

10. Zieve D, Henochowicz SI: Medline Plus: A service of The U.S. National Library of Medicine National Institutes of Health. http://www.nlm.nih.gov/medlineplus/ency/article/003519.htm.

11. Williams P, Sewell WAC, Bunn C, Pumphrey R, Read G, Jolles S: **Clinical Immunological Review Series: An approach to the use of the immunological laboratory in the diagnosis of clinical allergy.** *Clin Exp Imunol* 2008, **153**(1):10-18.

12. Tjon JM, van Bergen J, Koning F: **Celiac disease: how complicated can it get?** *Immunogenetics* 2010, **62**(10):641-651.

13. Schmitt WH Jr, Leisman G: **Correlation of applied kinesiology muscle testing findings with serum immunoglobulin levels for food allergies.** *Int Jnr Neurosci* 1998, **96**(3-4):237-244.

Appendix B

Quick Reference Guides

For nutritional supplements and personal-care products that we use or recommend and for other resources, go to www.theprotocolforhealth.com

Here are the guidelines and key points from this book:

THE SEVEN SOLUTIONS

Outlined in Chapter 1 and detailed in Chapters 4 through 10.

1. Eliminate Chronic Intestinal Infection and Prevent Its Recurrence

After eliminating chronic intestinal infection, its recurrence is much less likely if strong stomach acid is maintained while following the rest of the Protocol. Stomach acid is maintained by taking zinc with HCl daily and by reducing physical stress by adhering to the six following solutions. In a period of extra stress or illness, it may be necessary to increase the amount of HCl taken with zinc. (See Chapter 4, zinc section of Chapter 7, and comments below).

2. Avoid Common Food Irritants

Avoid corn, soy, dairy, gluten, and problematic additives. See pages on those foods and personal care products. (Chapter 5 and the following pages).

3. Keep Blood Sugar Stable

Consume adequate protein frequently in the busy part of your day and be mindful of the quantity and timing of caffeine or other stimulants. (See Chapter 6, Blood Sugar Stability - Adrenal Support Guidelines and the following pages).

4. Eat and Absorb Simple Nutrients

It's difficult or impossible to fully absorb and utilize adequate vitamins, minerals, and other key nutrients without maintaining strong stomach acid and supplementing with some or all of the Basic 9 supplements. (See Chapter 7 and www.theprotocolforhealth.com).

5. Avoid Excess Carbohydrates

Most people do best on a low-carb Paleo diet. (See Chapter 8, Chapter 5—Simple Foods Diet, and the following pages).

6. Walking or Sustained Mild Aerobic Exercise

Walk (or some similar continuous activity) for forty minutes, five or six days per week. This is perhaps the simplest, most important thing we can do for our health. (Chapter 9).

7. Resolve Residual Muscle Injuries

With the previous six factors in place, most old injuries resolve spontaneously or can be identified and cleared with manual muscle testing or other skilled bodywork. (Chapter 10).

★★★

Don't settle for a partial solution. Persistent symptoms point to an unresolved component in the big picture of your health. Every issue resolved makes the body stronger overall. Stay healthy and be prepared for possible adversity.

Not addressing any one of the seven pieces can undermine the entire Protocol. Weak stomach acid is the most common obstacle to return for my established patients. It is often caused by excess caffeine, lack of mild aerobic exercise, inadequate or infrequent protein, and/or eating too many carbs.

While most supplements have little to no benefit, the Basic 9 *actually* achieve noticeable results *when they are actually absorbed*. In case of nausea soon after taking the Basic 9, taking more HCl will likely resolve the nausea and facilitate absorption. If you experience the sensation of a burning stomach immediately after taking HCL, take less HCl or stop it entirely. If the burning is significant, seek professional help.

In general, the more the Protocol is followed, the less HCl is required, but there are factors beyond our control.

As long as HCl does not cause a burning stomach immediately after taking it, the dose should be increased by two tablets under the following conditions; cold or flu, leg cramps or other signs of poor (mineral) absorption, heartburn after a meal that is within the guidelines of the Protocol, an extended period of higher than normal physical or emotional stress, or to prevent symptoms with the occasional consumption of foods that fall outside the Protocol that have previously caused you negative symptoms.

These are general guidelines for people of average health without complicated conditions. If your health is more compromised or complicated, or you have significant symptoms, or these guidelines create negative symptoms, seek professional help.

ZINC DEFICIENCY—INTESTINAL INFECTION FLOWCHART

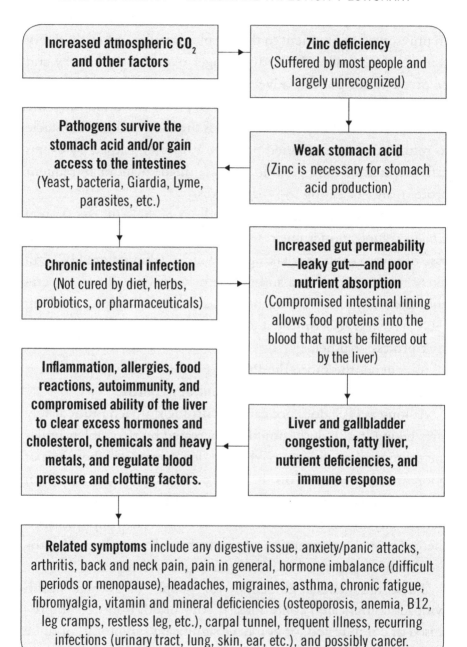

Increased atmospheric CO_2 and other factors

→ **Zinc deficiency** (Suffered by most people and largely unrecognized)

↓

Weak stomach acid (Zinc is necessary for stomach acid production)

→ **Pathogens survive the stomach acid and/or gain access to the intestines** (Yeast, bacteria, Giardia, Lyme, parasites, etc.)

↓

Chronic intestinal infection (Not cured by diet, herbs, probiotics, or pharmaceuticals)

→ **Increased gut permeability—leaky gut—and poor nutrient absorption** (Compromised intestinal lining allows food proteins into the blood that must be filtered out by the liver)

↓

Liver and gallbladder congestion, fatty liver, nutrient deficiencies, and immune response

→ **Inflammation, allergies, food reactions, autoimmunity, and compromised ability of the liver to clear excess hormones and cholesterol, chemicals and heavy metals, and regulate blood pressure and clotting factors.**

↓

Related symptoms include any digestive issue, anxiety/panic attacks, arthritis, back and neck pain, pain in general, hormone imbalance (difficult periods or menopause), headaches, migraines, asthma, chronic fatigue, fibromyalgia, vitamin and mineral deficiencies (osteoporosis, anemia, B12, leg cramps, restless leg, etc.), carpal tunnel, frequent illness, recurring infections (urinary tract, lung, skin, ear, etc.), and possibly cancer.

Simple Foods Diet

A variation of a low-carb Paleo or ketogenic diet. An approximation of the pre-agriculture diet.

Foods to Eat:

- Meat, eggs, and vegetables. Meat should be mostly nitrite/nitrate-free, additive-free, or better quality. While grass-fed and organic products are ideal, for those on a tight budget, conventional meats and vegetables are better than grains as far as personal health is concerned. The other pieces of the Protocol improve the body's ability to eliminate added hormones and pesticides.
- Nuts and seeds in moderation and only if there is no intestinal irritation or diarrhea. Safest to avoid peanuts because of mold and other factors.
- Nut butters in moderation—almond, cashew, sunflower, etc. (not peanut).
- When reducing carbohydrates, you will probably need to increase fat consumption for energy production. You may need to eat more of these foods: butter, avocados, olives, coconut, soy-free mayonnaise, fatty meats, and oils. Cheap oils often include problematic chemical solvents.
- Goat cheese, water buffalo cheese. Goat milk or goat yogurt are okay but are higher in sugars than cheese.
- Coconut milk (canned). Coconut milk in a carton usually contains too many additives.
- Vegetable juice and sauce (carrot, tomato, etc.). Watch out for citric acid and ascorbic acid (usually made from corn).
- Sea salt, spices, mustard, and types of vinegar that are free of additives, MSG, and white vinegar (usually made from corn).
- Possibly organic unsweetened almond or other nut milk. Cheap products often contain chemical solvents, corn, or soy. Those with especially compromised health may need to avoid nuts.

Optional:

- Caffeine in moderation and only within one hour after eating protein. If you drink decaffeinated coffee or tea, it should be "water process" and/or organic and treated as caffeine.
- Wine, but even organic sulfite-free wine usually contains added corn or chemicals. It's difficult but possible to find wine without problematic additives.
- Distilled spirits (tequila, Scotch and Irish Whiskey, and some brands of vodka test okay) in moderation and best after protein.

Keep Carbohydrates to a Minimum. Avoid most sugar and starch. If you exercise a lot or if your energy crashes with fewer carbs, you may need to add some **reasonable carbs** when starting this diet, such as half a sweet potato, some goat yogurt, or a little fruit. If it's difficult at first, understand it gets easier with the rest of the Protocol in place. Once your condition has stabilized and/or you're about two months into the Protocol, you might experiment with the reintroduction of more carbs, but most people find they feel better with minimal carbs.

Intestines: If you have diarrhea or intestinal discomfort, don't eat spicy foods, raw vegetables, salads, nuts, or seeds (unless ground smooth, maybe), or berries with seeds, and peel any fruit. When the intestines resolve, some of these foods can be reintroduced.

Foods to Avoid:

- Corn, cow dairy, soy, and gluten (wheat, spelt, barley, and rye); ideally, not even in small amounts.
- Grains and pseudo-cereal grains, such as quinoa, amaranth, and buckwheat. Bread, pasta, crackers, oatmeal, cookies, tortillas, chips, and other foods made from grain.
- High-carb, gluten-free products made from rice or other carbs and xanthan gum (usually made from corn).
- Sweets or products made with sweeteners except for possibly

stevia. NOW brand powdered stevia tastes better than most stevia and it tests fine.
- Fruit, fruit juice, and dried fruit, but small amounts may be used for flavoring or as described above in carbs.
- Rice, legumes (beans, lentils, and peas), potatoes, and sweet potatoes, but small amounts might be okay.
- Non-organic milk substitutes with sugar, allergens, or solvents (soy, rice, almond, oat, hemp, etc.).
- Highly processed meats, energy/protein bars or drinks, but they might be okay if low carb and additive/allergen-free.
- Sweet soda, beer, energy drinks, sweet wine, bourbon, gin, and sweet alcohol (rum, liqueurs, etc.).
- Flax, blue-green algae, chlorella, spirulina, wheatgrass, reishi mushrooms, and powerful herbs such as ashwagandha, wormwood, valerian, etc.

Eat plenty and often to control cravings. Eat breakfast within thirty minutes of rising. Don't go more than three hours in the busy part of the day without eating protein. You might need to set a timer. After a few weeks, you might try reintroducing a single serving size portion of **reasonable carbs** (see above) at every other meal or less.

When you eat carbs, you will crave more for a day or two. If you eat more carbs during that time, your craving may get out of control. Eating excessive carbs makes a low-carb diet suddenly boring and unappealing.

Mild aerobic exercise increases tolerance and decreases cravings for carbs.

Learn to cook. Look online or for Paleo/keto cookbooks, recipes, and mail-order food or prepared meals. Cooking on a BBQ is easy—no clean-up. Get help from friends, family, support groups, and online blogs.

Try the above Simple Foods Diet for two months. Treat it as an experiment, be creative, and feel better!

Cow Dairy Avoidance

Avoid foods made from cow's milk: milk, cheese, yogurt, sour cream, cream, whipped cream, half and half, cottage cheese, cream cheese, ice cream, whey (milk protein), casein, caseinate, lactalbumin, lactose, and colostrum.

The following foods are likely to contain cow dairy: milk chocolate, custard, pudding, cream soup, sauce, salad dressing, gravy, batter, bread, breaded foods, muffins, cake, cookies, protein drinks, energy bars, candy bars, most desserts, and flavored chips or flavored popcorn.

Problematic dairy alternatives (avoid): soy products (milk, ice cream, cheese, etc.), non-dairy creamer (made with hydrogenated oils and other chemicals), and cow dairy products with added lactase enzyme (still contains milk proteins).

Surprisingly, the following foods sometimes contain cow dairy (check ingredients): margarine, soy cheese, imitation dairy products, non-dairy creamer, salami, lunch meats, sausage, hot dogs, liverwurst, and pâté.

Foods that are not cow dairy (usually okay to eat): eggs, calcium lactate, cocoa butter, cream of tartar, and lactic acid.

Dairy products that are usually okay: most **butter** and ghee (clarified butter) from cow's milk (because the large proteins are removed, except for one brand of popular organic butter which leaves in more of these proteins), and **goat** and **water buffalo** dairy products (even though they contain lactose). Best to avoid sheep dairy products, but they may be okay for some.

Products that are okay for most patients who are cow dairy sensitive (Some of these are high sugar but could work as an occasional treat. Check ingredient labels and watch out for added chemicals or other possible food allergens/irritants): goat milk products such as goat milk, goat yogurt, various goat cheeses (jack, cheddar, gouda, brie, blue, etc.), condensed goat milk, goat cream cheese, goat ice cream (LaLoo), goat whey protein powder, water buffalo mozzarella, organic alternative milks (almond, hazelnut, hemp, rice, etc., but check ingredients), coconut milk (canned not boxed, good in coffee and recipes), dark chocolate bars and chocolate chips (watch out for soy), and coconut milk ice cream (Coconut Bliss).

GLUTEN AVOIDANCE

Avoid grains containing gluten: wheat, barley, rye, spelt, and anything made from these grains including bleached flour, unbleached flour, all-purpose flour, whole wheat flour, unspecified flour, sprouted wheat, wheat berries, wheat bran, wheat germ, wheatgrass, wheat gluten, bulgur, couscous, tabouli, farina, hydrolyzed wheat protein, modified food starch, semolina, durum, triticale, and Kamut. Oats in the U.S. are usually contaminated with gluten during storage and transport. There are gluten-free oats and Irish oats that are probably okay.

The following foods normally contain gluten (some come in gluten-free versions, which may or may not be healthy food): pasta, noodles, bread, croutons, stuffing, cake, pastries, cookies, crackers, communion wafers, pretzels, crepes, breakfast cereal, pizza, falafel, candy, licorice, play dough, gravy, marinade, lunch meat, hotdogs, jerky, soy sauce, beer, anything breaded and fried (fish, chicken, calamari, etc.), malt, caramel color, MSG (monosodium glutamate), modified food starch, hydrolyzed vegetable protein, supplements, drugs, and more.

Gluten-free products are usually made from other high-carbohydrate foods, such as rice, garbanzo beans, potatoes, quinoa, buckwheat, sorghum, tapioca, etcetera. While these may be okay for an occasional treat, frequent consumption is an obstacle to optimal health. More problematic is that many gluten-free products contain ingredients usually made from corn (xanthan gum, citric acid, ascorbic acid, white vinegar, alcohol, baking powder, corn oil, etc.) or soy (soy lecithin, soy sauce, vitamin E, tocopherols, soy oil, etc.) or cow dairy products (powdered milk, whey, cream, etc.). If you know you don't react to corn, soy, or cow dairy, you might choose to eat those foods, but most people either react to them and are unaware of the reaction or will probably start to react to those foods at some point. It's best to avoid these ingredients. More companies now make better products with just a few simple ingredients and/or less sugar.

Soy Avoidance

Avoid foods made from soybeans: tofu, miso, edamame, tempeh, seitan, soy sauce, soy aminos, soy oil, vegetable oil, soy protein, soy nuts, soy milk, soy sprouts, soy lecithin (which may just be called lecithin), tocopherols or alpha tocopherols (vitamin E), MSG (monosodium glutamate), glycerin, hydrolyzed vegetable protein (HVP), and textured vegetable protein (TVP).

Foods that usually or possibly contain soy: mayonnaise, margarine, movie theater "butter," ice cream, salad dressing, cheap olive oil, artificial cheese (often used on cheap pizza), teriyaki, sushi roll sauces, jerky, BBQ sauce, carob products, meat substitutes, most chocolate bars and chocolate chips, protein/energy/candy bars or drinks, and most corporate, restaurant, prepared, and deep-fried foods.

Non-food sources of soy: skin lotion, face cream, sunscreen, chapstick, shampoo, conditioner, fabric softener, diapers, laundry detergent, and some facial tissue.

Soy-free products: soy-free chocolate bars and chocolate chips (Equal Exchange is probably the most widely available), cocoa powder, coconut aminos (soy sauce substitute), mayonnaise made from canola, safflower, or avocado oil, and miso made from garbanzo beans or other non-soy beans. Lemonaise mayonnaise contains vinegar that appears to be corn-free.

Corn Avoidance

Avoid corn-based foods: whole corn, corn on the cob, corn chips, popcorn, corn tortillas, cornbread, cornmeal, polenta, tamales, corn masa, corn starch, corn syrup, high-fructose corn syrup, corn oil, corn cereals, corn-breaded food, corn sugar, hominy (pozole), grits, corn flour, sorbitol, and corn alcohol, which is sometimes added to herbal tinctures, beer, wine, liquor, etc..

Watch out for products that usually or possibly contain corn (check ingredients): candy, baking powder, vanilla extract, herbal extracts, CBD oil, ethanol, alcohol, grain alcohol, jam, canned tomato products and other vegetables, vinegar, white vinegar, distilled white vinegar, ketchup, mustard, pickles, soda water, tonic water, most sweet drinks in a jar, fruit juice in a jar, vegetable juice in a jar, bourbon (always at least 51 percent corn), vodka (not always corn), gin (always tests poorly), soy milk, most vitamins and supplements, vitamin C, ascorbic acid, ascorbate, citric acid, citrate (often combined with minerals in supplements), vitamin E, tocopherols, vitamin A, retinyl palmitate, caramel color, artificial sweetener, xylitol, breath mints, baker's yeast, fructose, glucose, dextrose (often in table salt), maltodextrin, xanthan gum (in gluten-free products), glycerin, powdered sugar, and sugar (as an ingredient can be corn sugar, beet sugar, or cane sugar), and most corporate, restaurant, packaged, deep-fried food.

Non-foods that may contain corn: chewing gum, pharmaceuticals (over the counter and prescription), paper cups coated with cornstarch, adhesive on envelopes and stamps, body powder, clothes starch, soap, shampoo, conditioner, toothpaste, and deodorant.

Corn-free products - while they do exist, they can be hard to find: xylitol (can be made from birch bark, but rare), stevia (NOW brand), xanthan gum (Bob's Red Mill—corn-free?), baking powder (Hain), mustard and BBQ sauce made with apple cider vinegar, pickles made without white vinegar, spaghetti sauce (Kirkland organic and others), and some distilled spirits (tequila, Scotch and Irish Whiskey, and some special vodkas).

BLOOD SUGAR STABILITY—ADRENAL SUPPORT GUIDELINES

The goal is to maintain stable blood sugar and avoid spikes and crashes. When stability is achieved, the adrenal glands no longer need to compensate for these swings, and adrenal function usually normalizes.

- Ingest caffeine in moderation only* and only right after eating protein.
- Don't ingest caffeine before breakfast or more than one hour after eating protein.
- Limit physical activity before breakfast to less than the equivalent of taking a shower.
- Eat a minimum of fifteen grams** of protein within thirty minutes of rising in the morning.
- Don't go more than three hours after a full meal without eating a protein snack during the busy part of the day.
- Eating a protein snack (seven-gram minimum) buys you one-and-a-half to two hours before your next meal.
- Eat a minimum of fifteen grams* of protein at lunch.
- Continue frequent protein during the busy, active, stressful part of the day.
- Limit caffeine to one reasonable cup per day. If there is a second dose of caffeine, it should be small and only occasional.
- Know that as we age, we become more sensitive to caffeine.

- Consider 50/50 regular/decaf organic coffee. Decaf contains up to one-third of the caffeine.
- Avoid decaf, chocolate, and caffeine four-plus hours before bed to ensure better sleep.

Good sources of protein are meat, poultry, fish, and eggs. If your digestion and elimination are very good (no diarrhea or discomfort), you might include nuts or nut butters. Significant quantities of nuts may cause weight gain or digestive disturbance, and those with especially compromised health may need to avoid nuts. Goat or water buffalo milk products are good protein sources for most people but may cause weight gain. Most react negatively to cow's milk dairy products but don't recognize its symptoms. Avoid it for at least the first two months of the Protocol.

* If your condition is more advanced (diabetes, etc.), or you want to eat more carefully, you might eliminate caffeine and alcohol as well as most carbohydrates. However, it's better to include these things in moderation and succeed on the other more important aspects of the Protocol than to deprive yourself of caffeine and/or alcohol and be overwhelmed and give up.

** Fifteen grams of protein is equivalent to two extra-large eggs or a little more than two ounces of meat or goat cheese or four tablespoons of nut butter. Fifteen grams is a minimum. An individual's age, size, and activity might indicate two to four times that amount.

EXERCISE GUIDELINES

For the first month or two of following the Protocol for Health, the most important aspect of exercise is that it is not an obstacle to healing. Most people who exercise, exercise too hard or anaerobically, which in the long run may stress the body, raise cortisol, and cause illness, injury, burnout, and increased fat storage. Any activity which raises the heart rate too high or which cannot be maintained for forty minutes is anaerobic and leads to overtraining if there is not a sufficient aerobic foundation. Even yoga and aerobics classes are usually anaerobic.

People were designed to walk, but now we drive cars. When we exercise at too high a heart rate or focus on strengthening muscles (whether they are biceps or the "core") rather than strengthening the heart, lungs, and vasculature, we take the body further out of balance. Exercising at a low heart rate, at a sustainable activity like walking, running, swimming, biking, or on a machine that simulates these activities creates an aerobic foundation. Once this foundation is in place and is maintained, strengthening muscles with anaerobic training can be accomplished without pushing the body out of balance.

If you don't currently exercise and you don't have much energy, you might wait until your energy comes up to start exercising, but you might just start walking (or doing a similar light activity) at an easy pace and find that it increases your energy.

If you already exercise, consider how it is working. If you have health problems (injuries or pain, weight you can't lose, multiple colds and flu, or systemic health problems), your exercise may be part of the problem. For the next two to four months, tone it down. Ideally, stop any weightlifting, sprinting, "pushing" or activities that can't be maintained for forty minutes. What yoga posture can you maintain for forty minutes? Not many. If you do yoga or similar activity, it should either be set aside for a couple of months or done at 50 percent effort with no strenuous postures. Try walking or slow running. When you go uphill, slow down a lot.

Monitoring your heart rate during consistent sustained exercise is the key to exercise success. This is best done with a heart rate monitor with a chest strap (other more convenient types of monitors may be accurate enough), but you can get an idea of your heart rate by stopping during exercise to take your pulse manually. If you are ready to focus your attention on sustainable exercise, then follow the guidelines below developed by Dr. Phil Maffetone and/or refer to his work in *The Big Book of Health and Fitness* or at his website, philmaffetone.com. His technique may be used for overall health and/or for maximizing athletic performance. Many top athletes credit him for how they went from burnout to world-class.

How to calculate your maximum aerobic heart rate.

- Start with 180 points.
- If you have health complaints, take prescription medication, or you have not been exercising or you have been exercising too hard (from the perspective of this technique), subtract 10 points or more.
- Also subtract your age.
- This gives your maximum aerobic heart rate.

For example, if you are 50 years old and have a health issue or take a pharmaceutical, your calculation is 180 minus 10 minus 50 equals 120.

This means that your heart rate or beats per minute (BPM) should not exceed 120 while you exercise aerobically. In this case a range of 110 to 120 is the ideal maximum, but most of the benefit can be achieved even at 20 to 30 BPM slower. If you work with the maximum numbers, the first quarter of your exercise time would be gradually increasing to that number, and the last quarter would be gradually bringing your heart rate down.

Exercise like this for 30 to 40 minutes, three to six times a week depending on your condition. You may need to check with your medical doctor if you have a health condition. Eventually you might increase your maximum heart rate by 5 to 15 BPM or more, but plan on working at this rate for at least a couple of months. While it will probably seem too slow at first, give it a good try. You will get faster at the same low heart rate. For a thorough discussion of this topic refer to Dr. Maffetone's books or website. It makes sense and it works.

Index

A

acid blockers, 141
acne, 64, 81, 86, 92, 150, 215
acupuncture, 10, 179
 meridians, 32
adaptogens, 227
ADD/ADHD, 95, 153, 244
addiction, 149–50, 154, 209–10
 and depression, 209
 sugar, 149, 156
adrenal glands, 104–5, 108, 111–12, 118, 186–87
 fatigue, 16, 25, 104–5
 muscle association, 108, 227
Adrenal Support Guidelines, 106, 110, 186
aerobic exercise, 159, 164
 foundation, 160–65, 190, 202–3
 training heart rate, 161, 166–67
Agent Orange, 113
aging, 105, 113
agriculture, advent of, 19, 65, 76, 158, 163
AK (applied kinesiology), 21, 23, 26, 28, 235–37, 242–43
alcohol, 94, 107

alcoholism, 209
allergies
 food, 13, 75, 82, 94
 seasonal or environmental, 48, 58, 68, 83–84, 86, 118, 243
American Medical Association, 142
anaphylaxis, 75
Ancestral Health, 11, 117, 158
anemia, 17, 32, 44
ankle injuries, 133
 excessive swelling, 67
 fracture, 163
 frequent sprained, 67
anorexia (poor appetite), 114
antacids, 139, 141
antibiotic-resistance, 157
antibiotics, 49, 61, 157, 206
antidepressants, 209
anxiety, 124, 135, 188, 210–11, 214
appetite, poor, 105, 114, 117, 214
apple cider vinegar, 142
applied kinesiology (AK), 21, 23, 26, 28, 235–37, 242–43
arthritis, 58, 66, 215
 associated with diet, 49, 81, 109, 150
 rheumatoid, 204

ascorbic acid, 70, 94
ashwagandha, 127
asthma, 147, 243
athletic performance, 193, 217
   and hormonal birth control, 193
atmosphere, CO_2 and zinc deficiency, 43, 143
attacks, panic, 124, 210
autoimmunity, 30, 59, 204
   conditions, 8, 58, 86, 190, 204–5
autophagy, 116–17
Ayurveda, 11, 135

B

babies and children, 213
baby formula, 214
bacteria
   beneficial, 47, 51, 60, 146
   coliform, 63
   die-off, 46
   pathogenic, 17, 46, 58, 140, 145, 156, 158
bacterial infections, acute, 120
   reducing recurrence, 189
bad breath, 64
Barr, Stephen, 179, 230
beans, 80, 149, 196
   garbanzo, 90, 93
beats per minute (BPM), heart rate, 161, 166–67
Beaver Fever, 57
bedwetting, 214
beer, 80, 90, 94, 98, 108
   and corn, 94, 98
bellyaches, 214
betaine hydrochloride (HCl), 15, 61, 119–20, 123, 141, 196
beverages, alcoholic, 94, 107
biopsies, 86, 183
   celiac disease, 86
   liver, 198
Biost supplement, 119, 137

bipolar disorder, 95, 188
birth, 194–95
   control, hormone, risks, 193–94
   and intestinal infection, 213
Bitney Springs, 63
black walnut supplement, 60, 121
bladder, sensitivity, 136
   infections, 156–57
bloating, 118, 150, 202
blood
   building, 132
   clotting, 197
   count, 25
   pressure, 203
   tests, 53, 124, 196, 198
blood sugar, 103–4, 108, 111–12, 187
   elevated, 197
   instability, 16, 103
   lab tests, 197
   stability, 16, 104, 106, 112, 187, 225
body
   fat, 201
   odor, 64
bone
   density, 118
   growth, 130
BPM (beats per minute), heart rate, 161, 166–67
brain, 95, 138, 177, 188
   chemistry issue, 209
breakfast, 16–17, 80, 103–6
breath, bad, 64
burnout, 164, 166, 203
burping, 64
bursitis, 66
butter, 85

C

caffeine, 16, 78, 107–8
calcium, 45, 123–26, 128–29, 135, 138–39
   supplements, 125, 129–30, 132, 241

cancer, 9–10, 48, 54, 76, 145–46
  colon, 61
  lung, 145–47
Candida, 46, 57
  diets, 60
carbohydrates (carbs), 19, 74, 79, 105, 108, 149–50
  addiction, 149, 156
  and illness, 156–58
  managing craving, 80, 152, 155–56
  and pancreas, 227
  reintroduction, 79
  See also low-carb Paleo diet
carcinogens, 147
cardiovascular system, 159, 162
carpal tunnel syndrome, 205
carrageenan, 101
casein, alpha S1, 19, 74, 81
CBD oil, 94, 100
celiac disease, 48, 86–87.
  See also chronic intestinal infection
cell division, 45
chemical irritants, 49, 76
  elimination, 7
  exposure, 33, 119, 147, 192
  as ingredients, 85, 100
  protection, 136
  in supplements, 18, 100, 124, 127, 129
  in wine, 79
children('s)
  and babies, 213
  health issues, 152, 157, 213
chiropractic, 10, 36–37, 59, 96–97, 180
  adjustments, 10, 36, 175, 234
    non-force, 36
  subluxations, 36
chlorella, 80, 127
chocolate
  and migraines, 207
  and sleep, 107, 208
  and soy, 70, 91, 93

cholesterol, 49, 197–98
chondroitin sulfate, 121
chronic
  fatigue, 44, 57, 123, 205
  pain, 8, 30, 59–60, 175
  stress, 105
chronic intestinal infection, 13–14
  and absorption, 134
  asymptomatic, 58
  and autoimmunity, 204
  and back pain, 30, 50, 54, 174–75, 219
  causes, 18, 47, 139
  and gut permeability or leaky gut, 48, 115
  and hypersensitivities, 49, 66, 75, 101, 147
  increased prevalence, 30, 59
  ineffective treatments, 60–61
  laboratory testing, 51
  and liver and gallbladder, 53, 121
  and lung infections, 146
  and Lyme disease, 206
  muscle testing for, 57, 60
  related to most health issues, 62
  treating with enzymes, 52
  types, 46, 57
  versus dysbiosis, 47
citrate, 132
citric acid, 33, 78, 94–95
  as a preservative, 68
  in supplements, 124
    and personal care products, 100–101
coffee, 16, 78, 107–8
  decaffeinated, 78, 208
colds, avoiding, 156, 165, 214
colic, 214
colitis, 48, 58.
  See also chronic intestinal infection
colostrum, 60, 84, 121
concussions, 217–18

congestion
    lung, 146
    sinus, 81
constipation, 51, 58, 121, 132
    and magnesium, 132
COPD, 145
core strength exercises, 175–76
corn
    avoidance, 98
    effects, 25, 95, 224
    as endocrine disruptor, 188
    and mental conditions, 188
    reaction
        lab tests, 72, 87
        muscle tests, 32, 74
cortisol, 104–6, 108, 111–12, 164
    and adrenal fatigue, 187
    and blood sugar, 104, 111
    and physical stress, 187
    and sleep, 208
COVID-19, 146–47, 157
cow's milk. See dairy
cravings, 80, 152, 154–55, 202, 210, 224
Crohn's disease, 48, 58. *See* also chronic intestinal infection

D

dairy
    allergy and sensitivity, 65, 68, 75, 81
    alternatives, 69–70, 74, 85, 242
    avoiding, 84
    buffalo, 74, 85
    calcium, 129
    goat, 19, 74, 77, 81–82, 85
    and headaches, 177
    lactose intolerance, 82
    and low back pain, 83, 174
    muscle tests, 74
    sheep, 85
    study, low back pain, 84, 233

decaffeinated coffee or tea, 107
deficiencies. *See* nutritional deficiencies
degeneration, arthritic, 109
dehydration and low back pain, 30, 32, 174
delayed puberty, 45
demonstration video, 24
deodorant, 99, 188
depression, 45, 70, 111, 188, 209
    postpartum, 195
dermatitis, 66. *See also* eczema
dextrose, 97, 99
diabetes, 76, 107, 190, 197, 203
    type 1, 190
    type 2, 190
diarrhea, 47, 81, 121, 132, 147
    basic dietary guidelines, 79
    chronic, 58
    in the developing world, 45, 146
    travelers,' 140 *See also* chronic intestinal infection
digestion, 15, 112–14, 145
    complaints, 46–48, 120–21
    of intestinal infection, 47
    red meat, 140
    and stress, 15
digestive enzymes for chronic intestinal infection, 15, 55, 146
digestive system paralysis, 62
disc herniation, 97, 175
diverticulitis, 58
drinking alcohol, excessive, 209
drugs, 6–7, 10–11, 61, 128, 142
    antacid, 141
    birth control, 194
    cholesterol, 174, 197
    intestinal side effects, 61
    mood-altering, 111
    prescription fatalities, 142
    side effects, 199
dust, 70, 136, 147
dysbiosis, 47, 49, 145–46
dysmenorrhea, 191, 215

E

ear infections, 156–57
eating, protein, 106, 113
   red meat, 77, 98, 119, 140–41, 169, 171
eating disorders, 114
Ebola, 157
eczema, 65, 81, 187, 214
eggs, 19, 72–74, 107
   sensitivity, 72, 95
elbow, 96
   repair, 217
   tennis, 96, 188
electromagnetic fields (EMFs), 210
elevated blood pressure, 203
emotional stress, 15, 59, 105, 164, 187
endocrine
   disruptors, 188
   system, 188
endurance, 124, 129
energy, 149–50, 165, 209–10
energy work, 179–80
Enzyme Defense supplement, 55–56
enzyme protocol, 51–52, 55, 143, 152, 198
enzymes, in red meat, 171
esophagus, 141, 143
estrogen, 54, 135, 195. *See also* hormone regulation
exercise, 19, 79, 152, 159–60, 164–65
   aerobic, 159, 164
   anaerobic, 163, 189, 202–3
   classes, 226
   core-strength, 10, 175
   high-intensity, 117

F

facial
   pain, 176
   tics, 188
fasting
   glucose tests, 197
   intermittent, 105, 114, 116, 118
fatigue
   chronic, 44, 57, 123, 205
   muscle, 129–30
fat intake, 202
fat-loss, 201
fats (dietary), 78, 154, 202
feet and hands, cold, numb, 92, 205
female hormone issues, 191
fiber, vegetable, 52
fibromyalgia, 44, 205
fish, 107
flax, 80, 127–28
flu, 150–51, 156
   and children, 213
   and exercise, 165
   and stomach acid, 62, 139
   and sugar, 189
folate, 132
food
   additives, 16, 94–95, 155
      undisclosed, 100
   allergies, 49, 71, 204, 243 *See also* food reactions
   challenge, 71
   irritants, four, 16, 68, 70, 72, 74, 76, 218
   and babies, 214
   and Lyme disease, 206
   and migraines, 176, 207
   poisoning, 15, 47
   and antacids, 139, 141
   and chronic intestinal infection, 146
   proteins in blood, 44, 48, 54, 66, 115 *See also* leaky gut
   sensitivities. See food reactions
   subsidized, 16, 33, 72
food-based supplements, 18, 120

food reaction(s)
  corn, 16, 65, 93–94, 96–99, 188
    See also corn
  dairy, 65, 68, 75, 81
    See also dairy
  extreme, 75
  gluten, 16, 72, 79, 86–89
    See also gluten (wheat)
  lab tests, 71, 87
    gold standard, 71
  muscle tests, 73
  nuts, 73, 75, 107, 192
    See also nuts
  soy, 16, 65, 68, 71–72
    See also soy
  spectrum, 72
foot
  arch support, 130
  pain, 123, 130, 201
fractures, 119, 138
fruit, 19, 149

G

gallbladder, 48, 115, 135
  attacks, 48, 53
  cleanse, 198
  clearing hormones, 192
  congestion, 48, 52, 120
gallstones, 48
garbanzo beans, 90, 93
gastroesophageal reflux disease (GERD), 142
gastroparesis, 58, 62
genes, disease-causing, 7
genetic modification (GMOs), 76
genetics, 7, 37
  and blood pressure, 204
  a non-diagnosis, 215
GERD, 142–43
geriatric muscle mass, 113
Giardia, 46, 57–58
gin, 80, 99
ginkgo biloba, 127
glands
  and corn and soy, 87, 95, 177
  and shoulder issues, 173
glucose
  from corn, 99
  elevated on low-carb diet, 197
gluten (wheat), 65, 70, 72, 79, 86–89
  avoidance, 88
  lab tests, 72
  and migraines, 207
  muscle test, 87
  prevalence of reaction, 88
  related conditions, 86
  spelt, barley, rye, 88
  types of reaction, 86
goat dairy products, 74, 81–82, 85
Goodhart, George, 230
grain alcohol, 94
grains, 19, 74, 76–77, 79, 149
growing pains, 129, 214
growth, poor, 45, 57, 129
guar gum, 101
gut bacteria, 14, 47, 147
  and lung issues, 145
gut-lung axis, 145–46

H

hair, thinning, 45, 64, 135
halitosis, 64
hand paralysis, 205
hands and feet, cold, numb, 92, 205
HCl, betaine, 15, 61, 119–20, 141
  See also stomach acid
headaches, 44, 46, 68–69, 176–77
  and blood sugar, 104
  and cow dairy, 69, 81
  and intestinal infection, 58
  and liver, 52, 56
  and smoke, 136
  and soy, 91
  tension, 27, 54

healing
    and cortisol, 187, 218, 233
    wounds, tissues, and zinc, 45, 116
healthcare, 5, 8, 18, 22, 40
heart, 19, 124–25
    arrhythmias, 124, 135, 210
    attack and magnesium, 124
    disease and cortisol, 164
    and exercise, 165
    and magnesium, 131
    and minerals, 124
    rate, aerobic, 19, 159–62, 164–67
heartbeat irregularities, 124, 135, 210
heartburn and reflux, 121, 124, 140–41, 144
heavy metals, 49, 54, 115, 135
hemorrhoids, 104
herbal tinctures, 94
herbs, powerful, 80, 121–22, 128
    and sleep, 207
herniated disc, 97
Herxheimer reaction, 46
hip pain, 83, 110, 135, 173, 191
    replacements, 109
hormones
    balancing, 192, 225
    and cortisol, 187
    imbalance, 44, 58, 184
    insufficiency, 195
    lab tests, 196
    menopause, 118
    regulation
        female, 45, 54, 187, 192
        male, 45, 54, 187, 191, 195
    synthetic, 125, 183, 192–94, 215
household products, 99, 188
hunger, constant, 202
hydrochloric acid, 15, 61, 119–20, 141
    See also stomach acid
hypersensitivities, 8, 72, 75
hypertension, 203
hypothyroidism, 205

I

IBD (inflammatory bowel disease), 48, 58. See also chronic intestinal infection
IBS (irritable bowel syndrome), 32, 47, 58. See also chronic intestinal infection
ICAK (International College of Applied Kinesiology), 26, 28
illness
    avoidance, 156
    chronic, 8, 39, 72, 82
    and cortisol, 203
    frequent, 44, 214
    and sugar, 157
immune system, 46, 48, 147, 156, 169, 204
infants, 213
infections
    colds, influenza, viruses, bacteria, 156
    in general, 156
    intestinal, 46
        See also chronic intestinal infection
    lung and lower respiratory, 146
    recurring, 70
    sinus, 81, 156–57
infertility, 215
inflammation, 34, 48–49, 65–66
    and acute injuries, 66
    and headaches, 176
    joint, 204
    and lungs, 145
    reducing, 155, 162, 205
inflammatory bowel disease (IBD), 48, 58. See also chronic intestinal infection
influenza, 147, 156
injuries, 20
    acute, 66
    chronic, 59, 67, 160
    from exercise, 160, 164

repetitive stress, 60, 205–6, 217–18
  specific treatment, 138, 169
  and sports, 217, 219
insomnia, 207
insulin, 189–90
intermittent fasting, 105, 114, 116, 118
International College of Applied Kinesiology, 26, 28
intervertebral disc herniation, 97, 175
intestinal
  conditions, 47
    See also chronic intestinal infection
  flora, 47, 60
  infection. See chronic intestinal infection
  permeability. See leaky gut
iodine, 134, 138, 185–86
  and shoulder weakness, 135, 173
  thyroid and soy, 186
Irish Whiskey, 99
iron supplement, 132, 135, 138
irritable bowel syndrome (IBS), 32, 47, 58. See also chronic intestinal infection
irritants, 70
  unidentified, 192
IUD (intrauterine device), copper, 194
IVF (in vitro fertilization), 195

J

jaw issues, 95, 177, 188
joint pain, 181, 187, 204, 236

K

kelp supplement, 91, 134, 185
ketogenic diet, 18, 77, 152, 155
kidneys, 32, 115
  and low back pain, 83, 174
kids' health issues, 152, 157, 213

knee pain, 16, 104, 110, 224
  replacements, 109

L

lab tests
  alternative medicine, 183
  chronic intestinal infection, 51, 57, 61
  effects of the Protocol, 197
  food reactions, 71–72, 88, 126
  hormones, 183
  limitations, 71–72, 74, 82, 87, 197
  minerals, 18, 125
  while taking enzymes, 198
  zinc, 126
lactation, limited, 62, 194
lactose intolerance, 57, 81–82, 84–85, 238
laundry detergent, 93
leaky gut, 44, 48–49, 66, 115
  and autoimmunity, 204
  and dietary protein, 141
  and food allergies, 75, 101
  and the immune system, 156
lecithin (soy), 91, 93
lectins, 49, 73
Lee, Royal, 55
leg cramps, 68, 124, 135, 214
  restless, 32, 44, 135
  weakness, 133
legumes, 74, 80, 149, 158, 189
L-glutamine, 60, 121
libido, low, 135, 195
ligament(s), 118, 175
  laxity, 16, 104, 130
lip balm, 91
liver
  and cancer, 54
  eliminating toxins and waste products, 48, 54, 115, 195
  enzymes elevated, 54, 198

fatty, 48, 54, 198
filter congestion, 48
and gallbladder support, 15, 48, 53, 120
and head to mid back pain, 27, 170, 176
and hormone regulation, 54, 184, 192, 202, 204
and low testosterone, 195
muscle association, 26, 54, 170
longevity, 19, 160
Lovett Brother Relationship (chiropractic), 96
low-carb Paleo diet, 18, 77, 154, 189
lungs, 19, 117, 145–47, 159–61, 163–65
conditions, 145, 147
microbiome, 1, 30, 146
Lyme disease, 157, 206
post-treatment, 46, 62
lymphatic system, 145

M

macronutrients, tracking, 154, 203
MAF (maximum aerobic foundation test), 162
Maffetone, Phil, 166
magnesium, 119, 125, 131–32, 135
and constipation, 132
and heart disease, 124–25
and shoulder weakness, 173
supplements with corn, 101, 124
malabsorption and acid blockers, 141
malaria, 45, 157
male hormone issues, 195
maltodextrin, 99
manual muscle testing, 11, 22–26, 28, 31, 33, 185
baseline, 22, 26, 28, 31, 237, 239
carb tolerance, 151
exercise load, 151
food reactions, 73

intuitive, 29
vitamin and mineral deficiencies, 119
maximum aerobic function test (MAF), 162
mayonnaise, 91, 93
meat, 19, 74, 77, 154–55, 202
non-organic, 76
reaction to, 73
red, 77, 119, 133, 140–41, 169, 171
meditation, 209
melatonin, 127, 208
menopause, 54, 118, 187, 192
menstrual
cramps, 68
cycles, difficult, 54, 191, 215
mental clarity, 152, 213, 224
conditions, 95, 188, 226
meridian system, 26
pulse points, muscle testing, 53
metabolic syndrome, 190
Metagest supplement, 139
metals, eliminating, 49, 54, 115, 135
metronidazole, 61
microbiota, 14, 47, 145, 190
microtrauma, repetitive, 60, 67
migraine headaches, 176, 206–7
mild aerobic exercise, 224, 226
milk
See dairy products (cow)
goat, 74, 81–82, 85
nut, 78
minerals, 45, 99, 124–26, 134, 208
absorption, 124, 139
deficiency, 17, 119, 128, 211
and anxiety, 210
symptoms, 123–24, 135
food source, 134
fulvic, 134
ionic, 134
optimal levels, 45
poor absorption, 18, 45
and sleep, 208

miso, 91, 93
  from garbanzo, 93
mold, 70, 78
morning sickness, 195
mouth sores, 45, 49, 92
MS (multiple sclerosis), 205
MSG (monosodium glutamate), 78, 90, 93
mucous membranes, 136
multivitamins, 18, 91, 94
  studies, 122
muscle
  cramps, 132
  fatigue, 130
  injuries, 20, 119, 170, 174, 177, 180
  mass, 113, 202
  spasms, 27
  testing. *See* manual muscle testing
  weakness, 2, 5, 24, 26, 28–30
  work, myofascial, 20, 169
muscle-organ/gland association, 26
muscles
  gastrocnemius (calf), 108
  gluteus maximus (glute), 135
  gracilis, 108, 174
  latissimus dorsi (lat), 151–52, 170, 173–74, 176, 189, 219, 233
  pectoralis major (pec), 27, 54, 170
  psoas major, 30, 83, 174–76, 233, 236
  quadratus lumborum, 236
  sartorius, 174
  scalenes, 102
  sternocleidomastoid (SCM), 170–71, 177
  subscapularis, 131
  supraspinatus, 95, 188
  tensor fasciae latae (TFL), 50, 175
  teres minor, 92, 135, 185
  tibialis posterior, 130
  upper trapezius (trap), 27, 58, 69, 151, 170, 177
mustard, 78, 94, 98–99

N

narcolepsy, 62, 207
nausea, 113, 123, 140, 144, 195, 222
neck pain, 27, 59, 150–51, 170, 190
nerves, pressure on, 97, 205
nervous system
  and B12, 132
  guiding care, 82, 88, 126
  and zinc, 138
neurotransmitters, 121, 183, 209
newborns, 213–14
nightmares, 129, 214
nightshades, 49, 73
NSAIDs (nonsteroidal anti-inflammatories), 66
nurses, 152, 159–60
nutrient absorption, 34, 112–13, 123, 135, 196
  insufficient, 126
nutritional deficiencies, 17, 120, 128, 138, 202
nuts, 19, 73–75, 77–79
  nut butters, 28, 107
  nut milk, 78
  and scalenes, 102
  sensitivity and allergy, 73, 75, 102, 107, 172–73, 177, 192

O

oatmeal, 79, 108, 149
obesity, 190, 201
odor, body, 64
  breath, 64
oils, 78, 94
  canola, 101
  CBD, 94, 100
  cheap, 78, 138, 177
  cod liver, 136
  essential, 94
  hydrogenated, 85

omega-3 fish, 121
palm, 101
vegetable, 91
opioid drugs, 59–60, 160
osteoporosis, 17, 32, 123, 125, 129, 215
overtraining, 152, 156, 164, 219

P

pain, inflammatory, 66, 82
Paleo, diet, 19, 74
　flu, 149
pancreas, 141, 152, 170, 174, 189–91
panic attacks, 124, 210
paralysis
　of digestive tract, 58, 62
　of hands, 205
parasites, 17, 46, 122
parasympathetic nervous system, 113
pathogens, 12, 46–47, 51, 145–46, 204
　ingested, 15, 17, 46, 63, 140–41
peanuts, 78
pelvic pain, female, 188
personal care products, 87, 99
pesticides, 49, 76–77
pharmaceuticals, 128, 141–42. *See also* drugs
physical stress, 15, 105, 141, 164
pickles, 94, 98–99
picky eaters, 214
Pilates, 189
pituitary, 95, 188, 195, 197–98, 209
placebo, 10, 36, 61
plantar fasciitis, 123–24, 130, 218
pneumonia, 45, 145–47
poison oak, 70
pollen, 70, 136
potassium, 134
potatoes, 19, 74, 76, 149
pregnancy, 45, 194–95, 215
preservatives, 16, 87, 91, 94–95
probiotics, 47, 49, 60–61, 121

pronation, shoes, 130
prostate, 188, 195, 197
protein
　digestion, 141
　drinks, 227
protein/energy/candy bars, 93
proton pump inhibitors, 141–43
protozoa, 17, 46, 140
PSA (prostate-specific antigen), 188, 197

Q

quinoa, 79, 90

R

rashes, 33, 214. *See also* eczema
red meat, 77, 119, 133, 137, 140–41, 169, 171
reflex points, 22–23, 49–50, 73
　neurolymphatic, 185
reflux, 140–41, 144
reishi mushrooms, 80, 127
repetitive stress injury, 206
reproductive systems, 135, 191
restless leg syndrome, 124
retinyl palmitate, 99, 136
rheumatoid arthritis (RA), 204
rice, 79–80, 89–90, 149
rotator cuff, 25, 92, 95, 131, 135, 173, 185
running (slow), 224, 226
rye, 79, 86, 88–89

S

salad dressing, 85, 93
salt
　and blood pressure, 204
　and corn, 97
　table, 99

saltwater pools, 161
schizophrenia, 45
scoliosis, 176, 216
secondary sensitivities, 71–72, 101
sensitivities, 76–77, 82, 136. *See also* irritants or food reactions
sesame oil, 135–36, 174, 191
sexual function, 135
shampoo, 91, 93, 99
sheep dairy products, 85
shellfish, 73, 75
shin splints, 218
shoes, flat, 130
shoulder pain, 95, 135, 172, 185
SIBO (small intestine bacterial overgrowth), 46, 57
Simple Foods Diet, 77
skin
    conditions, 8, 57, 91, 135, 150, 215
    lotion, 70, 91, 93
sleep, 10, 16, 107, 110, 207–9
    apnea, 201
    and fasting, 117
    and stimulants, 107
smell, decreased sense, 45
smells, hypersensitivity, 114, 214
smoke, wood, sensitivity, 136, 147
smoking, 147
    quit, 209
snacks (protein), 104, 106
soap, 99, 188
soy
    avoidance, 92
    lecithin, 70, 90, 93
    oil, 91
    in personal care products, 91
    reaction, 16, 65, 68, 71–72
        and carpal tunnel syndrome, 205
        and endocrine issues, 188, 195
        laboratory testing, 71, 87
        muscle testing, 74
        symptoms, 91
        and thyroid, 186

spirulina, 80, 127
spitting up, new borns, 214
sports
    drinks, 94
    injuries, 60, 172, 206
    performance, 162, 218
sprains and strains, 66, 169–70, 172
    ankles, 133
Standard Process supplements, 55
starch and sugar, 19, 79, 103–4, 149, 151, 189. *See also* carbs
steroid drugs, 66
stevia, 80, 99, 222
stiff joints, 135
stimulants, 105, 208
stomach (empty)
    and caffeine, 16, 103, 105, 116
    and carbs, 104
    and exercise, 118
stomach
    symptoms, 120
    ulcer, 144
stomach acid
    and apple cider vinegar, 142
    and heartburn and reflux, 121, 124, 140–41, 144
    and mineral absorption, 17, 130, 139
    and overall health, 143, 195, 214, 225
    and pathogens, 17, 46, 64, 139
    production, 15, 17, 141
        muscle testing, 25
    and stress, 105–6, 127
    supplement, 15, 123, 140
    suppression, 141, 143
    and zinc, 15, 123, 127, 138
        medical study, 138, 142
strength
    athletic, 161–62, 193, 217
    core exercise, 175–76
    training, 162–63
strep throat, 156
stress
    and absorption, 62, 139, 141, 144

and autophagy, 116
  and cortisol, 127, 187, 208
  emotional, 111
  emotional vs. physical, 15, 27, 106
  and exercise, 117, 164
  and fasting, 114
  greatest, 159
  liver, 54
  organ and glandular, 48, 105, 188
    causing muscle weakness, 27, 32, 104, 174, 227
  pancreas, 170, 189
  physical, 111
  and sleep, 208
Strong, Evan, 218
study of dairy and low back pain, 233
sugar and starch, 19, 79, 103–4, 149, 151, 189
  addiction, 149, 156
  See also carbs
sun exposure, 137
sunscreen, 91, 93
superfoods, 127–28, 227
supplement list of the Protocol
  Biost, 119
  calcium lactate, 128
  cod liver oil, 136
  Enzyme Defense, 55–56
  kelp, 134, 186
  magnesium, 132
  Metagest, 139
  sesame oil, 135
  vitamin, B12, 133
  Zinc A.G., 139
  Zymex II, 55–56
supplements
  absorption vs. utilization, 45
  Basic 8 or 9, 119–20, 128, 196, 225
  betaine hydrochloride (HCl), 123, 138, 144
  and corn and soy, 71, 87, 91, 94, 99–100, 188
  for deficiencies, 17, 119, 126, 204–5
  effective, simple, 18, 120–21, 123–24
  vs. foods, 131
  for inflammation, 121
  interfering, 127
  for intestinal infection, 55–56
    prevention, 62
  liver and gallbladder, 53
  minerals
    calcium, 125, 128. *See also* calcium
    fulvic acid, 134
    iodine and trace minerals, 134, 185. *See also* iodine
    ionic minerals and dissolved rocks, 134
    iron, 133. *See also* iron
    magnesium, 132. *See also* magnesium
    zinc, 138. *See also* zinc
  muscle testing, 21, 28, 73, 120, 127
  poor ingredients, 18, 124, 227
  poorly absorbed, 45, 122, 183–84
  potential unrecognized, 45
  red meat enzyme, 171
  synthetic vitamins, 16, 70, 91, 94, 98–99, 136
  thyroid, 185
  used in the Protocol, 120, 247
  vitamin(s)
    A and low back pain, 30, 174
    B12, 57, 132, 208
      absorption, 123
    C, 95
    D (hormone), 121, 125, 137
    E, 90–91, 93
sweeteners, 80, 99
sympathetic nervous system, 112, 127

T

tendons and tendonitis, 66, 104, 118

tennis elbow, 96, 188
tension headaches, 27, 54. *See also* headaches
testosterone, 45, 54, 187, 195. *See also* hormone regulation
TMJ (temporomandibular joint), 95, 177, 188
tocopherols, 90–91, 93, 99–100
tofu, 91, 93
tomatoes, 49
　canned, 94
toothpaste, 33, 99, 188
trauma, physical, 119, 138
　emotional and physical, 58–59, 105, 209
travelers diarrhea, 47, 139–40. *See also* chronic intestinal infection
triglycerides, 197
tropical diseases, 46. *See also* chronic intestinal infection
turmeric, 66, 121

U

ulcerative colitis, 48, 58. *See also* chronic intestinal infection
urinary tract infections (UTI), 44, 156–57

V

valerian root, 127
vanilla extract, 94
vegetables, 19, 74, 77, 104, 154–55
　canned, and corn, 98, 188
　cooked, 52
　and deficiencies, 43
　non-organic, 76
　raw, and intestines, 79
　reactions, 73, 77
　starchy, 154
vegetarian, 69, 140, 184, 227

vertebra(e)
　C1 and L5 association, 96
　first cervical and pituitary, 95, 177, 188
　lumbar, 174
　relationship, Lovett Brother, 96
video demonstration, 24
vinegar, 78, 93–94, 98
　apple cider, 99, 121, 142
　balsamic, 100
　white, 94–95
viruses, 17, 140, 156, 158, 189
vision
　double, 188
　and zinc, 45
vitamins. *See* supplements, vitamin(s)
vodka, 99
vomiting, 113, 123, 140, 144, 195, 222

W

walking, sustained, 224, 226
weakness, muscular, 12–13, 20–21, 24, 26–27, 31
weight
　inability to gain, 113
　losing too much, 202
　trying to lose, 115–17, 156, 165, 201–2
whey (cow), 84, 90
white vinegar, 94–95
wine, corn and chemicals, 78–79, 94, 98
women, pregnant, 113, 194
World Health Organization, 45, 126, 157
wormwood, 60, 80, 121, 127
wrist conditions, 67, 96

X

xanthan gum and corn, 89–90, 94, 99–100
xylitol and corn, 99

Y

yeast overgrowth, 17, 46, 58, 61
yoga, 12, 164–65, 189–90

Z

zinc, 15, 17–18, 43, 45–46, 123–24,
    138–41, 143
  absorbing, 15, 17, 139, 196
  and absorption of other nutrients,
    15, 123
  and atmospheric changes, 43
  and cerebrospinal fluid, 138, 177
  and heartburn and reflux, 121, 124,
    140–41, 144
  and immunity, 157
  medical study, GERD, 142
  and newborns and children, 213
  and prostate, 196
  and stomach acid, 15, 17
  and symptoms of the head and
    neck, 177
  usable, 139
Zinc A.G. supplement, 139
Zymex II supplement, 55–56

About the Author

Dr. Matt Archer lives in Northern California with his wife and two daughters. He and his family raise their own farm-fresh eggs, grass-fed lambs, and tend their orchard, vegetable garden, and trail network to help create a connected, daily celebration of life. Matt's other loves include forest management, amateur naturalism, skiing, mountain biking, kayaking, woodworking, hiking, scuba and freediving, international travel, backcountry exploration, and the inner work of being happy.

Made in the USA
Monee, IL
01 February 2021